THE
MIND
MANUAL

DR ALEX GEORGE

THE MIND MANUAL

Mental Fitness Tools for Everyone

ASTER*

This book is dedicated to Carly Cook and Harry Grenville, my dear friends and colleagues, without whom none of this would be possible.

First published in Great Britain in 2023 by Aster,
an imprint of
Octopus Publishing Group Ltd
Carmelite House
50 Victoria Embankment
London EC4Y 0DZ
www.octopusbooks.co.uk

An Hachette UK Company
www.hachette.co.uk

Distributed in the US by
Hachette Book Group
1290 Avenue of the Americas
4th and 5th Floors
New York, NY 10104

Distributed in Canada by
Canadian Manda Group
664 Annette St
Toronto, Ontario, Canada M6S 2C8

ISBN 978-1-78325-490-3

A CIP catalogue record for this book is available from the British Library.

Printed and bound in Italy

10 9 8 7 6 5 4 3 2 1

Publisher Stephanie Jackson
Art Director Jaz Bahra
Senior Editor Alex Stetter
Design and Illustration Abi Read
Copy Editor Lucy Bannell
Photographer Andrew Burton
Props Stylist Agathe Gits
Props Assistant Nicole Theodorou
Food stylist Lizzie Kamenetzky
Hair and make up Victoria Barnes
Production Manager Caroline Alberti

Photographs on pages 6, 25 and 202: Courtesy of Dr Alex George

All reasonable care has been taken in the preparation of this book but the information it contains is not intended to take the place of treatment by a qualified medical practitioner.

Before making any changes in your health regime, always consult a doctor. While all the therapies detailed in this book are completely safe if done correctly, you must seek professional advice if you are in any doubt about any medical or mental health condition. Any application of the ideas and information contained in this book is at the reader's sole discretion and risk.

CONTENTS

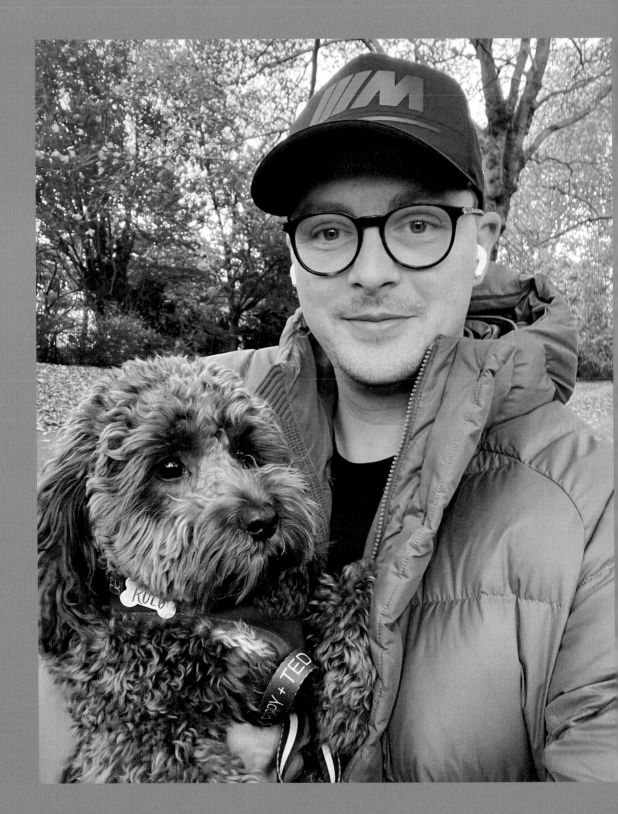

INTRODUCTION

How are you?

No really, how are you?

I'm assuming that picking up a book called *The Mind Manual* means you're interested in your mental health, that you'd like to be proactive about it. You may be doing quite well at the moment, but want to learn more about how to keep things that way. Or perhaps you're finding life a little challenging and would like some tools to help you to regain a solid footing. Either way, you're in the right place. Welcome.

If you're anything like I was when I first started focusing on my mental health, you'll be wondering, 'Where do I start?' 'What can I do?' 'Why don't I already know this?'. We are taught many useful life skills at school, but unfortunately mental fitness is not one of them. Instead, this area of our health has been kept under wraps, as if a mental health crisis doesn't affect us humans, which means that – when we feel the wobble of things going south – we believe there must be something 'wrong' with us. If we were never taught that life's challenges will affect our mental health, then we will naturally judge ourselves when they do.

Where do you start? Here. In these pages. This manual will teach you to find a baseline of peace in your life, which can help you to manage the highs and lows that will arrive. It will teach you to use tools to build a life that feels full, not one that just checks all the boxes. It will teach you how to stretch your mental muscles regularly, just as you would your physical ones. It will teach you that you are not alone on this journey. It will teach you how to thrive.

THE FIGHT FOR MENTAL FITNESS

Whether you're reading this book right now from a place of calm or crisis, I hope you find some help within its pages. I wrote this book for a number of reasons, but, essentially, I wanted it to help readers to find a balance in their lives. When I wrote my first book, *Live Well Every Day*, I wanted to offer an overview of health and the 360° approach we could take to feel healthier. This book is different. It is about mental fitness and the peace that it can bring.

I have written *The Mind Manual* because I want to change the conversation about what mental fitness is and how we should approach it. While the national conversation on mental health has seen an improvement in services and how we talk about times of crisis, we rarely (if ever) talk about the everyday effort that is required to keep our mental health in check.

There are countless books, TV shows and streaming documentaries about how to manage your physical fitness. What to eat, how to move, who to follow – there is a guru for everyone. On the whole, we understand that in order to keep ourselves free from disease and injury, we must take care of our physical fitness and do so regularly and consistently. We know our vices and we have also been taught how to counter them with healthier choices, so that the overall balance sheet of our physicality leans towards health. But we don't do the same when it comes to our mental fitness. I want to change that.

I like to think of mental health as a spectrum. At one end, we have depression, anxiety and all the mental illnesses that make us feel miserable. Let's consider that end as set at minus five on the spectrum. On the other end of the spectrum, we have happiness, joy, excitement. These would be set at plus five. The centre point of the spectrum is set at zero. This zero is the equilibrium we feel when we're at peace, it is the baseline we should aim for in life. You might be surprised to hear me say that peace, not happiness, is the goal. I believe that it is more realistic to aim for peace than to expect happiness 24/7. I believe that, for good mental health, we should aim to move away from living with the sharp peaks of highs and deep troughs of lows, and instead ebb and flow more calmly on either side to keep on an even keel.

This is what mental fitness means to me. It's the middle ground. It's looking at the balance sheet of all that you do in a day, a week, a month, a year, and assessing whether your mentality is healthy or unhealthy. It's knowing your vices – your unhelpful mental habits – and learning how to counteract them. It's using tools to push yourself when you simply 'don't feel like' making healthier mental choices, just as we have strategies to motivate us when we don't want to go to the gym. It's essentially creating a personalized toolkit of all the things you need to keep yourself at peace, then actively applying them on a daily basis, not just when you're in crisis.

WHY ME? WHY NOW?

If you've been following me, you'll know that I've been through a particularly rough few years. In July 2020, my 19-year-old younger brother Llŷr unexpectedly took his own life. As you can imagine, it was like a tsunami of pain hit our family, sweeping each of us up into our own journey of grief. Llŷr's absence left a gaping hole in my life and, at first, I just didn't know how to cope.

Even before his death, after years of struggling with my own anxiety, I had been creating a 'mental health toolkit' that could help others build up their mental dexterity. And after Llŷr passed, while I was grieving and growing, I developed this even further and became more convinced of the need to spread the idea of mental fitness as far as it could possibly reach. Not just as a tribute to Llŷr, but as a tribute to the mental anguish I have faced in life, both before and since his death.

After I began to understand my own grief, I reached out on my social platforms, talking more and more about the importance of mental fitness. In late 2020, the world was experiencing grief on so many levels, as lockdown after lockdown kept us indoors and away from the people we loved. Depression and anxiety rates increased, many sought help from their doctors and I looked on as so many people struggled to maintain balance in their lives. I wanted to help in whatever way I could.

In February 2021 I was given the opportunity to do more, when I was named as the British Government's Youth Mental Health Ambassador. In this volunteer role, I combine my clinical expertise as an emergency care doctor with my personal experience, to champion children's mental health and to shape policy on improving support for young people in schools, colleges and universities. This role has allowed me to meet people up and down the country, to hear their stories and learn from them about what they need.

Later in 2021, for the fundraiser BBC Children in Need, I filmed a documentary called *Our Young Mental Health Crisis*. It explored the impact that mental illness has on young people's lives and what education can do to help ease pressures before they occur.

Month by month, the more I learned and shared about mental health education, the more opportunities came my way. I grabbed each one, with the goal of getting the mental fitness message out there as far and wide as I could. Writing this book is the culmination of that aim. It's me gathering everything I've learned academically, professionally and personally about mental fitness to create something tangible for you to hold on to. A life raft that you can use to support you when you need it most.

HOW TO USE THIS BOOK

This book is broken down into four parts. I like to think of each one as building on the last, in the same way you think of foundations being laid in a building, before the ground, first, then second floors can go up. The goal is to help you to establish your baseline, to know what peace feels like to you. And then to offer advice and tools to help you maintain that as much as possible.

PART ONE looks at how mental health has become increasingly topical in recent years, how we have been talking more about it and allowing ourselves to feel more of what we actually feel, instead of how we 'should' feel. This section will show you that you are part of a growing community of people who are tired of the judgmental narrative and want to learn how to help themselves. From there, we'll look at how to figure out where your baseline is. What normal feels like for *you*, specifically. It's good to get in touch with recognizing your own needs, so that you can best support yourself when issues arise.

PART TWO explores the seven universal truths that I want you to cling to. When you are moving towards the negative side of your mental fitness baseline, experiencing depression or anxiety, your brain can try to convince you of all manner of untruths. It can tell you things you'd never believe when life feels good. It can make you think that you're not enough, that nobody cares, that you'll never be happy again, that you don't matter. The seven truths are here to support you when your mind is telling you lies like this. They are true no matter how you're feeling, so you can rely on them even when you feel less like yourself. These seven truths are: Connection is your superpower; Sleep will save you; Boundaries are beautiful; Mistakes are a must-have; Stress is the enemy; You are enough; Happiness is an inside job. Swear by these truths and they'll keep you afloat.

PART THREE focuses on the foundations of mental fitness. In this section, we'll explore five different areas of life. These include what you eat and drink, how you release stress from your body, how much you move, how to talk out your thoughts and how to approach the medical side of things. You can set yourself up to win by making sure you're maintaining strong standards within each of these areas.

Throughout these first three sections, you will also find four recurring features, flagged up under the following headings: My Experience, Challenge the Narrative, Take Action and No Time Like Now.

PART FOUR is your mental health toolkit, where you'll find a wide range of worksheets and activity tools to use. These can help while reading the book, but can also be used regularly in your day-to-day life to check in on how you're coping.

At the back of the book, you'll find a list of resources that can help you maintain your mental fitness. You'll find services listed that can help in crisis and others to assist you in maintaining calm, so you always know there is support for you when you need it.

Read this book as many times as you feel necessary. It's your mind manual, for your mental health. Your experiences are unique, so your journey will be too.

MY HOPES FOR YOU

One of the most important lessons I'd like to share from this book is that looking after your mental fitness means taking a 360° approach to your physical and emotional health. Living a life where you feel at peace 80 per cent of the time is a wonderful achievement, but you can't achieve that with a quick fix. It requires consistency and – yes – a little bit of work. I like to look at it this way: feeling miserable most days is an exhausting way to live. Life *feels* hard. So, although taking care of your mental fitness requires daily effort – which at times can involve hard work – the effect is that life *feels* really good. Pick your hard. I know which one I'd choose.

If I have done my job, you'll finish reading this book feeling empowered. You'll know that, no matter where you are on the mental fitness spectrum right now, you have the tools to reach a baseline of peace. You may not reach that centre point today or tomorrow, but you'll know that it's possible and what steps to take to get there.

If I have done my job, you'll feel so good most of the time that you'll want to pay it forward.

If I have done my job, together we'll help pull people out of pain into the life they truly want to live.

Your struggle is valid, no matter how many people have it 'worse' than you.

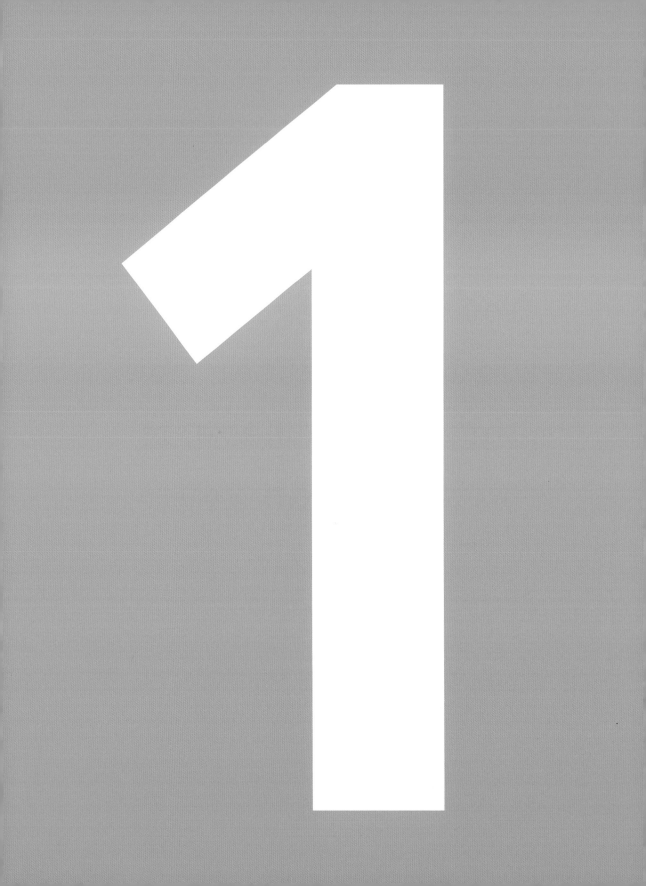

YOUR MENTAL HEALTH TODAY

YOU ARE
NOT ALONE

You don't need to struggle in silence.
You are part of a large community of people
making choices to improve their mental health.

You'd be forgiven for assuming that everyone in your peer group is breezing through life. Daily updates of happy faces on your socials – posting #goals or #blessed – can make us believe that we are the only ones struggling. That, somehow, we've failed at this adulting thing.

The truth is that the statistics prove otherwise. In England alone, one in every four people – 25 per cent of the public – experience a mental illness, such as depression or anxiety, every year. If you think about that for a minute, you'll realize that in a room of 20 people, 5 will likely be struggling. If I think back now to my class sizes at university, I realize that I wasn't alone in what I was going through. I was likely one of about 70 people – that's a lot!

If that number of people are living with mental illness, then it is more common than getting the flu (figures from just before the pandemic suggested that roughly 9 in every 100,000 people in the UK showed flu symptoms). Think about how much we talk about the flu and how common it is. Now consider how little we talk about mental illness and how much *more* common that is. That's shocking, isn't it?

You are part of a community of people who'd like a little extra help to find their baseline. Mental struggles are a natural part of life. We all face hurdles and challenges, we all get knocked down a few times in our lives. We are not robots, but living, breathing, mistake-making humans.

In this chapter, we will look at just how common mental health conditions have become. I want you to see that, if you find yourself facing one of them, it isn't something to berate yourself about. They are a common condition of living in a modern world.

THE PANDEMIC EFFECT

Since the pandemic of 2020, our lives have changed dramatically. I'm not talking about the physical changes – lockdowns or the need for vaccines – I'm talking about the habits we have now developed as a society. Habits that are exacerbating existing mental health conditions and making life that little bit harder, as if it wasn't already hard enough.

The effects of the pandemic are long-lasting, not just in terms of how we protect ourselves from infection, but in how we operate in our daily lives. Our social lives have been affected; our communities have dispersed. The pandemic saw many people migrate back to their home towns, out of cities, meaning that those left behind were faced with isolation. Our work lives have been turned upside down, as remote and hybrid working suddenly became the norm. And while many celebrate spending less time commuting, few factor in the mental cost of working from home, the blurred lines between your place of stress and your place of rest. Our wellbeing has been affected by these changes. External factors, which all made sense at the time they were enacted, have now led to a mental health crisis, in which people feel isolated, lonely, always-on … and yet entirely disconnected. Now, more than ever, we need to know how to find what peace means to us – and proactively work to include it in our lives.

TALKING ABOUT MY GENERATION

Millennials are those born between 1981 and 1996. The generation is characterized by technical savviness, fondness for transparency, inclination towards collaboration over hierarchy, adaptability to change and passion for learning. They are free-thinking and creative.

Generation Z, more commonly known as Gen Zs, are those born between the years 1997 and 2012. This generation is characterized as technical natives, who see diversity as the norm, are politically progressive, pragmatic and the most sociable generation yet.

Both these generations have traits that have been challenged by the pandemic. The collaboration that Millennials crave, and the socializing of Gen Zs, are both now in shorter supply.

More and more studies are focusing on the effects the pandemic has had on Gen Zs and Millennials. They show that those aged 18–40 across the world appear to be experiencing the same thing, that their emotional health and wellbeing have been greatly affected.[2] The certainty about their future that they possessed before 2020 has all but vanished. Instead, they are left with concern over their careers, the cost of living (nearly half are living pay cheque to pay cheque), the climate and the general state of geopolitical discord. To them, the future doesn't look as bright as it once did. No wonder that this has changed how they feel about life.

WHAT HOLDS US BACK?

Good physical and mental health are intertwined: one can't exist without the other and a balance between the two is key to wellbeing and happiness. But even the phrase 'mental health' is sometimes infused with a negativity that 'physical health' is not. Often, when people speak about 'mental health' what they really mean is 'mental illness'; too often 'mental health' is used in conjunction with the words 'issues' and 'problems'. This tendency to interchange the meanings has the result that, as far as a lot of the general public are concerned, there's no positive state for mental health. You rarely hear of people talking about being in good mental health, though they commonly talk about robust physical health.

Stigma is sticky, and takes a long time to dissolve. Thanks to the views of our great-grandparents, who lived through world wars, we've been handed down a belief that it's best to keep a stiff upper lip. To keep calm and carry on. This was to dispel the fear of being seen as weak, the concern that if – for some reason – we showed our human side, we would expose our underbelly to the enemy and be defeated. It was a fear of displaying vulnerability, that somehow we would be challenging our safety if we showed the least sign of that. But in the modern world, our resilience is not found in a grin-and-bear it attitude, but in a share-and-grow-from-it one.

Thankfully, stigma surrounding mental health is slowly falling away, but until it has gone completely, opportunities to have frank discussions are often limited. It helps when people in the public eye talk about their own experiences, so it is encouraging that celebrities such as Lady Gaga and Stormzy have come forward and spoken about their own struggles with depression, anxiety and post-traumatic stress disorder (PTSD). The thing to remember is that we all sometimes hit a bump in the road and we all need to ask for help when it happens. That doesn't mean we have failed or are 'less than' others, it just means we're human and we're alive. And that's a good thing.

You haven't yet experienced all of your happiest days!

MY EXPERIENCE

GRIPPED BY PANIC

Last year, I went away for a night to film a TV appearance in Manchester about the youth mental health charity HEADucation. I arrived at my hotel the day before the shoot, had some food and went to bed at a sensible time. I wasn't particularly anxious about the filming. It was live, but I was okay with that and I got to sleep with no problem.

At around 4:30am, I suddenly woke with a sense of impending doom, as if I was about to die. I was experiencing a panic attack. My heart was beating out of my chest, my skin felt as if it was on fire, I was finding it hard to breathe. I couldn't lie still, so I got up and paced around. I was feeling faint and the tightness in my chest made me want to scream out for help. I was in the hotel room alone, worried that it was too early in the morning to disturb anyone. Even then, as a mental health advocate, despite the advice I gave to others, I failed to contact anyone else. I struggled through it alone.

I tried out the tools I'd been sharing with everyone else, how to become present in the moment, to distract from the fear that had triggered the attack. I slowed down my breath and was mindful of each inhale and exhale. Then I used the Five Senses Technique (see page 162) to name items in the room, helping me to be more present and less in panic. The palpitations did eventually abate, but I couldn't get

back to sleep and still felt awful when the car came to take me to set a few hours later. Once I got there, I'd calmed down a bit and after speaking to the producers I felt normal again.

Fortunately, nothing like that has happened since, but it did have a huge impact on me. As an emergency care doctor, I think I'm pretty tough on the whole, but that experience really gave me a new perspective and appreciation for what people who struggle with anxiety issues go through. It made me think how terrible it must be if such experiences are part of your daily existence.

It's also a good example of how on the outside things might look okay, while on the inside all is not well. There I was, on live television, talking to teachers and pupils about how they can improve their mental health education, when just a few hours earlier I had experienced a full-blown panic attack.

I can pin the reasons for that particular episode down to overwork and a triggering few days. On my tour of schools around the country, I had visited my brother Llŷr's old school earlier that week, and that, no doubt, had affected me. But if I really unpick it, my acute anxiety was a culmination of everything you're going to read about in this book. Fear of failure, loneliness, impostor syndrome – they're all things that I've experienced in my life and, to a lesser degree, continue to experience.

EARLY INTERVENTION IS PARAMOUNT

When I was in the middle of my panic attack, having the tools I needed to calm myself down helped significantly. And while the attack came as a warning sign that I needed to make some adjustments, what I had to question was: 'Why did it come to that?'

Mental Health Foundation research has proven that early intervention is the best way to tackle a mental health crisis.[3] The idea is to spot signs or situations that may challenge a person's mental health, then step in to provide help before they reach a crisis point. For children and teenagers in the UK, this could take the shape of Early Support Hubs. They provide information, advice, guidance and access to evidence-based support, delivered by council staff and partner agencies. Children and teenagers can drop into these centres to access help for their mental health and wellbeing and they're also a community space, where people can feel like they belong. In my role as Youth Mental Health Ambassador, Early Support Hubs have been and remain a key ask to the Government in supporting young people's mental health.

As adults, we need to consider our own ways of approaching early intervention. We need to create our own form of support system. More than anything else, we need to be sure we have a number of options to reach out to in times of crisis. Of course, we may only need them on rare occasions, but knowing they exist prevents us from dipping too far into isolation. For me, that support system includes my family, a handful of really close friends, my doctor, my therapist and the range of tools I use on a regular basis to keep me balanced.

I've included everything I've learned about maintaining mental fitness in this book, so you should have your toolkits covered by the time you've finished reading it. You'll also learn who to reach out to and when. Just keep in mind that you should create a support system *before* you need it, not after. So start building it now.

Asking for help
is not a sign
of weakness,
it's a sign
of strength.

#POSTYOURPILL

Back to that hotel room in Manchester. Even though it hasn't happened again, I took that panic attack as a sign. So, I went to see my doctor and she prescribed a number of lifestyle changes, along with an antidepressant.

Since losing my little brother Llŷr, my increased workload and the pressures that came along with it had kept me from looking after certain areas in my life as well as I should. For a lot of people, me included, there are times in life when you get shaken, something happens and you fall out of sync with yourself. My medication keeps me balanced, so I can sort out those areas that need attention while still getting on with the day-to-day.

I think of these medications as fuel for the brain: they give you the energy to deal with those things that make your brain tired. They quieten the anxiety, which allows your mood to improve and gives you the mental energy you need to be yourself again. And because you feel better, you'll want to do those things that are good for you, such as exercising, eating well, engaging with your friends... all of which are hard to do when you're stuck in a difficult mental space. They help you get back on the right track.

There are many people who have mild or moderate depression or anxiety who would benefit hugely from medication. That said, there's a stigma attached to it, an idea that taking it – or having therapy – somehow prevents you from being successful and happy. I believe the opposite is true. It's this judgement and discrimination that inspired me to start the #postyourpill campaign on social media in 2021. I asked people to join me in taking a proud stance against medication stigma by posting a picture of themselves and their pills every month on social media, whether that be Instagram, Facebook, TikTok or Twitter.

People all over the world started sharing their medication stories and the hashtag shows that taking medication for mental wellness is in fact incredibly common. Thousands of people have already joined the movement, so the proof is in the posting! Hopefully, people struggling with feeling they are alone in taking medication will see that they're not.

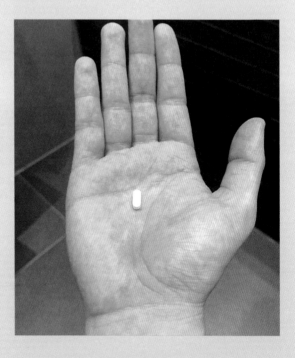

EMOTIONAL LITERACY

Although there have been massive improvements in the discussion of mental health in recent years, it's still a bit of an uphill struggle, particularly around the language used to talk about mental wellbeing. But happily, it seems that the younger generation are leading the way in improving that.

On my school visits, I've noticed that kids seem far more emotionally literate than previous generations. They're so open and compassionate. In fact, I think a big reason why we're seeing so many more referrals for issues with mental health in young people is because that age group can articulate themselves far more eloquently than us Gen Zs or Millennials can.

Words have power; the language we use *matters*. It's important to check in with yourself about words before you use them. If you are weaponizing words to tease others, based on perceived characteristics, then you've likely crossed a line. For example, if you mock a friend as 'schizo' because you think they are being paranoid about something, you are weaponizing your words. You may not mean to offend, but that doesn't mean you aren't offensive. Always consider your language before you speak.

Reducing the negative use of words creates a more positive space for those who are living with mental illness. It also allows us to celebrate the benefits of successfully dealing with challenges when they arise.

We should all be talking positively about how good mental health enables us to enjoy life to the full and experience peace, purpose and fulfilment. All of these things are well within our grasp.

One lexical change I really do want you to consider is when talking about someone who has taken their own life. People 'die by suicide' or they 'take their life', they do not 'commit suicide'. That expression dates back to a time when suicide was considered a crime: you 'committed' the crime of suicide. That law hasn't existed in the UK since 1961 and yet the expression remains. What this language does is frame this enormously challenging time for those involved in the person's life with the idea that what the person did (or tried to do) was morally wrong, to the point of criminality. And when you think about the cruelty of that for someone living with the legacy of a death, or an attempt to end their own life, you'll never use it again.

It's time to challenge the narrative. Every time someone in your circle chooses to use damaging language around mental health, ask for a reframe. Educate, don't shame. We want to keep the conversation as positive as possible so that we don't overcorrect to the point of stigmatizing again. Rewording yourself is a simple switch, but the more we do it on a daily basis, the more it will seep into the greater consciousness. Choose to be a voice of reason.

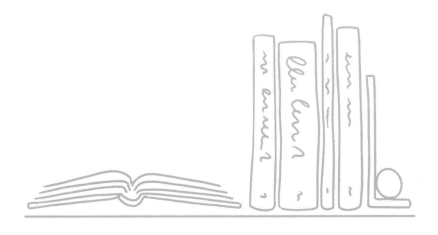

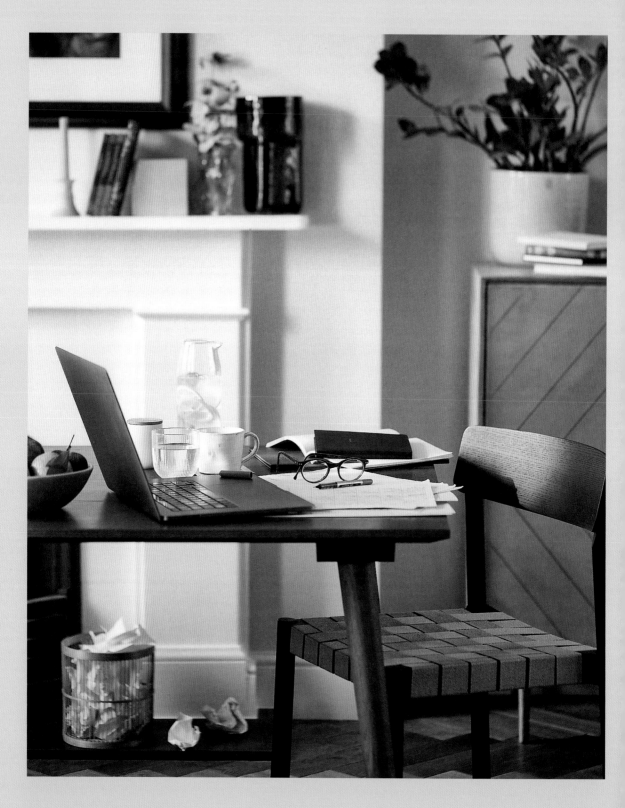

THE WONDER OF WATER

I want you to try this trick now, so that you have it ready when you need it most. The idea is that you go to the sink, grab a glass, fill it with water and drink the entire thing right there and then. Water is amazing for us, for hydration, for clarity, for detoxification, but what this trick does is activate many of our senses at once. Sight: you watch the water fill from the tap. Sound: you hear it as it pours into the glass. Touch: you feel the glass between your fingers, perhaps a little wet from splashes. Taste: you taste the water as you gulp it back. Smell: you can smell whatever else is going on in the room, as water's neutral scent forces us to extend our senses. Activating all these senses with one simple action will give you not just the physical benefits of hydration, but the mental benefits of being in the moment. Try it!

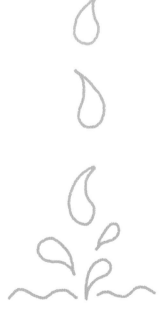

KNOW WHAT FEELS NORMAL FOR YOU

Understanding yourself is key to your mental health. Learn how to track your mood, so you know when support is needed.

How you feel on a daily basis really matters.

Life can be tough at times, of course, but overall you should be feeling like you love life and living. From where you're sitting right now, you might be thinking, yeah right, Alex! Who really loves life? Well, *you* should. No seriously, you should.

We know that mental illness runs under the radar. We know that society has created an environment where we don't talk about it, don't address it as an issue. Instead, we try to plaster over it by achieving the next goal, then the next goal, hoping that'll be the thing that – finally – makes us happy. We can learn to live with a certain 'meh'-ness about our lives. We feel as if it's all just a blur of grey. We get up every morning, head to work, whiling away the hours until we can return home again, before numbing ourselves with junk food or alcohol as we binge-watch a series on TV. We're coping, but we're certainly not thriving.

That's why it's important to assess where you currently are on the mental health spectrum. That one I was talking about in the introduction (see page 8). It's good to know where you are, so you can figure out where you'd like to be. And none of this has anything to do with external factors, but essentially how you feel about life. What do you feel now? And what do you *want* to feel in the future?

This chapter is about figuring out your spectrum: everyone is different. What feels like peace to me may feel challenging to you. What feels unpleasant to me may feel exciting to you. Everyone has their own personal taste that affects what they define as good, bad or ugly. Here, you'll learn to figure out what that looks like for you.

WHAT DOES GOOD MENTAL HEALTH FEEL LIKE?

Now you know there is no standard measure for good mental health. Some people can live and function quite happily with levels of stress and anxiety that others would find difficult to handle. Likewise, behaviours that in some would be disruptive can be the norm for others. Feelings such as anxiety, worry and low mood are experienced by most of us. The trick is knowing when those things tip over, moving from what's acceptable to you, to a situation that you can't bounce back from, then to a point where you need outside help.

According to well-respected US medical research centre the Mayo Clinic, when we experience good mental health, we should be able to:

- **Maintain personal or family relationships.**
- **Function in social settings.**
- **Perform at work or university.**
- **Learn at a level expected for our age and intelligence.**
- **Participate in other important activities.**

Let's look at this list a little deeper, to understand what such broad advice can mean on a personal level, and why each area should matter to our wellbeing.

Maintaining personal or family relationships is important because loneliness breeds depression. You are a creature of community, not isolation. When you feel connected to others, you will feel there is more value in life, that it is here to be shared. This may mean finding new people who you can feel connected to, if existing relationships are troublesome. Being engaged in healthy, connective relationships will make you feel as though you belong, as well as build your self-worth. They will support you and give you the opportunity to support others in return.

Our ability to function in a social setting is not just about being the life of the party. It's about how we deal with relationships and that is down to our self-worth and our identity. If you are comfortable around others, it is normally a sign that you are comfortable with yourself. Your self-worth is not tied into how others view you, instead you happily allow yourself and others to shine. This is the case for conflict in social settings too. How you deal with conflict says a lot about how you feel about yourself. If you handle conflict well, knowing that you cannot agree with everyone all the time, then you're likely to be feeling peace in your life on the whole.

While some of us can perform well at work or university even when we are living with mental illness, you could say we'd be white-knuckling our way through. When your life is in balance, you can perform with a sense of focus and calm: you are not reacting to events, but peacefully moving from task to task. How you handle the pressures placed on you says a lot about how close you are to burnout, or to overextending yourself.

No matter how old we get, we will never stop learning. People who are content know this. They don't see growth as something limited to their school days, but rather they allow themselves the space to learn at every stage of their lives. In fact, when you feel good about life, you want to learn as much as you can, because you like how it feels to stretch yourself. You see growth as a challenge, not a crisis.

One of the greatest signs of someone who is living a life that feels good is what they choose to involve themselves in. There are certain activities that we *have* to do to be functioning adults, such as pay the bills, clean the house or visit our family. And while these are obviously important, those who feel good about life add on extra activities for the sheer fun of it. They are full of energy for the life's little bonuses. They add joy and pleasure whenever they can – they seek it out. A life that feels good feels full.

ARE YOU FEELING GOOD RIGHT NOW?

Ask yourself these questions to find out if you are living with a sense of mental wellbeing. Where do you think you are on the mental health spectrum? For each question you answer positively, add one, as that's how you should be feeling when at peace. But for each question you answer negatively, subtract one, so that you find out where on the spectrum you're sitting right now. And whatever the overall picture looks like (if you're feeling particularly bad, you could end up with minus five), help is here. Just read on.

1. **Do you feel connected? Do you feel like you belong? Are you part of a community?**

2. **Do you play well with others? How do interactions with others make you feel?**

3. **How emotionally reactive are you at work/university? How do you handle pressure? How well do you think you're performing?**

4. **Do you seek out opportunities for growth? What new thing have you learned in the last month? Do you have plans to take on a new challenge?**

5. **Do you seek out pleasure and joy? Do you have the energy to add fun activities to your life? When was the last time you felt like you did?**

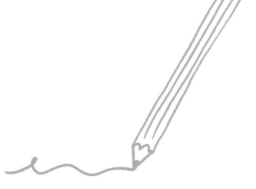

However good or
bad a situation is,
it will change.

HOW I KNEW I NEEDED HELP

When I had that panic attack up in Manchester, I had been close to burnout. Even though I knew the signs, the symptoms and even the tools that could head off a crisis, I hadn't put them in place to help myself. My brother's death and, after that, the pressures I put myself under, were enough to push me over the edge. But the seeds of my mental illness were planted long before Llŷr left us.

You could say that I grew up an anxious child. It's funny now that I write it out, as I now know anxiety is so common in childhood. For me, the anxiety was likely brought on by undiagnosed dyslexia and ADHD. When I went to school, the words on the board made no sense to me and I always seemed to find it hard to focus. I was told I was smart, but for some reason I seemed to find everything so much harder than my classmates. I overcompensated and my anxiety helped me to do this. Driven by fear of failure, I pushed myself in every area of my life. And if I was faced with a moment of panic, before a rugby match for example, my parents would say, 'What's the worst that could happen?' With that fear out of the way, I'd push on through and take on every challenge that I faced.

My parents definitely imparted some fabulous tools to help me overcome my anxiety in my school years, but it seemed to take on a life of its own once I moved out of home. Having missed out on med school on my first attempt, when I finally made it to Peninsula Medical School, I felt I had something to prove. I put my head down and burned myself out. I allowed my anxiety to take the driving seat and it meant that I led a rather lonely existence for the five years I was studying. Here I was, learning about how the body responds, while putting mine through the mill.

Before my panic attack in Manchester, I had been pushing myself again. Forcing myself to do more, help more, be better. Llŷr's death made me double down on my efforts to educate others on the importance of mental health, while I was ignoring the alarm bells ringing inside me. I have not had a panic attack since, but that's not the only thing that's changed. I've given my entire life an overhaul. I've really practiced what I preach. I've built up solid foundations for my mental good health and found my baseline. If nothing else, I'm proof that you can do it too.

SIGNS OF STRESS

Our physical health influences our mental health and vice versa. Here's a handy infographic that shows how anxiety and stress can affect our bodies. Experiencing any of these could be an indication that you may need to pay attention to an aspect of your mental health – and, of course, take action.

Heart palpitations.

Insomnia.

Constant headaches.

Tight, tense neck and shoulders.

Stomach issues such as cramps, nausea and loss of appetite.

Teeth grinding and aching jaw.

Pulsing or whooshing sound in your ears.

Hot flushes and sweats.

Always tired and fatigued.

Bitten/picked nails.

Other digestive issues, such as IBS.

Restless leg syndrome.

MEN AND MENTAL HEALTH

The tools in this book are for everyone, no matter their gender, but I do want to touch on men and mental health, because I feel that they've been conditioned even further than women have. The toxic, boys-don't-cry message of 'You must be tough', 'You must be strong', 'You must be resilient' robs men of everything that makes them human. There is nothing physiologically different about men when it comes to emotions. They experience the same feelings as women do. The difference is that society doesn't allow them to express certain emotions, or at least frowns on them when they do. And what is the worst thing a man can be called? Weak. To bypass that, many men avoid talking about their vulnerabilities.[4] And the statistics show that three times as many men as women die by suicide.

If this is you, I urge you not to become a statistic. Use this book to guide you to a place where you can open up about what you're going through. And if you know a man who you suspect may be struggling, I urge you to use the Ask Twice tactic. If you ask, 'How are you?' and you're met with the answer, 'Fine', ask again. Ask, 'How are you really?' They may answer you honestly that second time, they may not. But at least they will know that you care and that you're someone they can turn to if things get bad.

MENTAL HEALTH MOT

Now that you know where you sit on the mental health spectrum, wouldn't it be good to figure out which areas of life are working for you and which aren't? I like to use the Wheel of Life (see page 228 for more on this) to give myself a mental health audit every now and then. It's a coaching tool that you may have seen used to reach goals and targets in your professional life, but it can easily be applied to any audit you want to do.

Start by drawing a large circle on a page (or use the guide on page 229). Then divide the circle into eight even slices, by drawing four intersecting lines across the circumference. Now, I want you to add a different area of your life into each of the sections. Let's include Connection, Career, Pleasure, Health, Finances, Growth, Worth, Home. Now, assess each section of the wheel on a scale between zero and ten. The centre point of the wheel is zero and the outer edge is ten. You can add markings to indicate each rating between those points if you like. Now, working through each area, rate your satisfaction level with it on the scale. If you're thinking about 'Connection', how connected do you feel on a scale of zero to ten? Mark it on the wheel and colour in that segment from the centre point outward to where you made your mark. Try and use different colours for each segment, so that you can clearly see how you feel about each area. Colour in all the eight sections. When you stand back from your completed wheel, you'll see which area of your life is giving you the most satisfaction and the part that is offering the least. This will give you a clear indication of which part of your life needs a little work.

You don't need to do anything about these results right now, but use them as a guide while reading through this book. Now that you have those areas in mind, you'll find that the tools that can help with them will stand out more than they would have before.

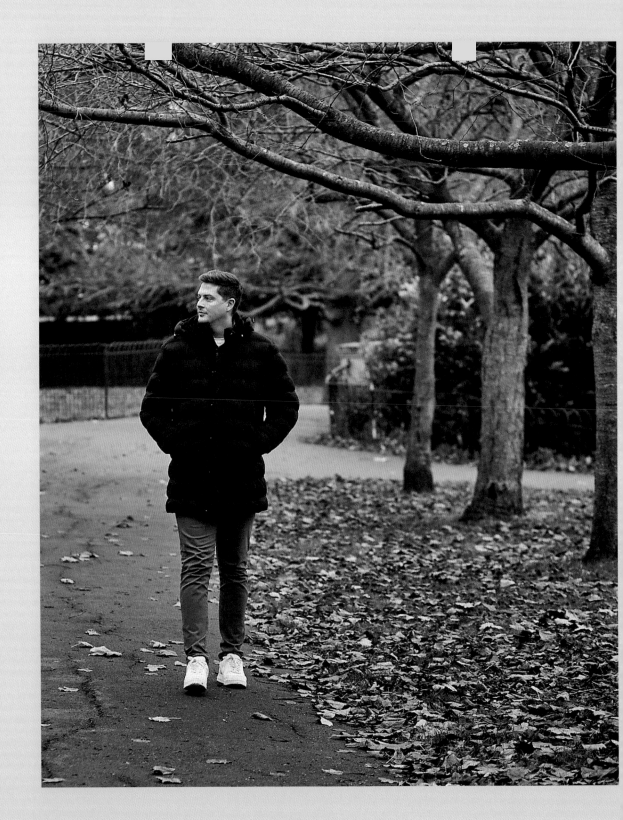

START TO STOMP

Rain or shine, I make sure to kick off my day with a daily walk, or, as I like to call it, a stomp! On the days where I miss it, my mood deteriorates. For me, there is just something so valuable in getting outside in the fresh air and moving those muscles. I know it's not always easy when your energy levels feel low and maybe the rain is beating down, but getting out there and doing even only a short stomp can work wonders for your mind. I love it so much that I even created a podcast called Stompcast, where I interview interesting people about their own mental health journeys while we stomp along together.

Now that you're at the end of Part One, I suggest you head out for a stomp. Get your body moving, breathe in the fresh air and appreciate the life that is happening around you. It will shift how you feel within minutes and even a 20-minute walk around the block helps. Try it!

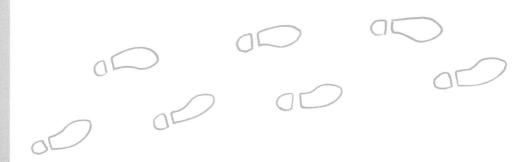

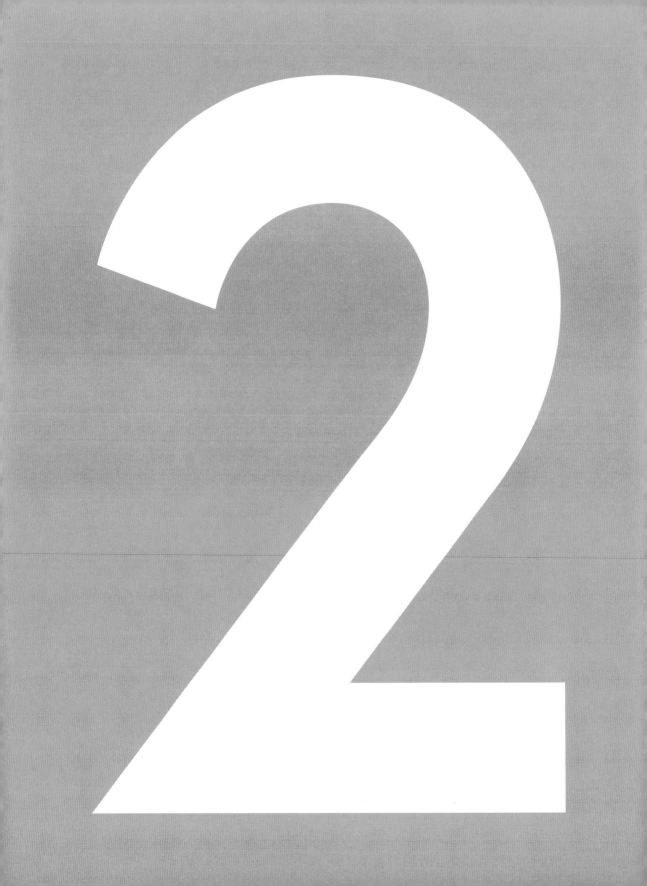

THE SEVEN UNIVERSAL TRUTHS

1

Connection is your superpower.

2

Sleep will save you.

3

Boundaries are beautiful.

4

Mistakes are a must-have.

5

Stress is the enemy.

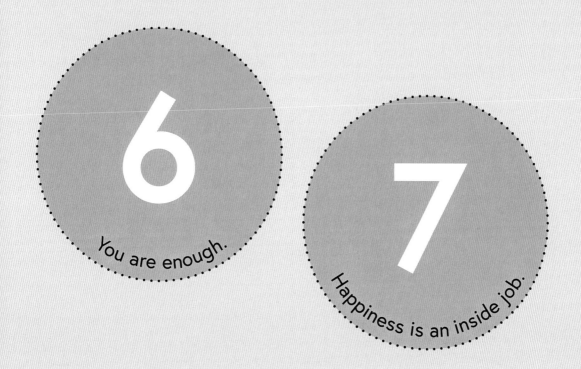

6 You are enough.

7 Happiness is an inside job.

Our brain can lie to us when it's in an unhealthy state. It can tell us that we're not good enough, that nobody cares, or that things will never get better. On an average day, we probably wouldn't heed these fabrications, but when we're feeling challenged and under pressure, we may start to believe that they're true. When that happens, I want you to remember the seven universal truths in this section. They will not change just because your mood does. Come back to them as often as you need, to remind yourself of the truth when your brain is trying to convince you otherwise.

CONNECTION IS YOUR SUPERPOWER

You are a social creature, one that thrives within a sense of belonging. Find out how your community can help you heal.

When your mental health is subpar, your brain will tell you that you are alone in what you are feeling. In fact, it will tell you that you are alone in this whole world and that nobody cares. That you are entirely isolated and left to manage your mental health without any external help. It will try to convince you that you are an island. That is not true.

As humans, one of our basic needs is to belong. It's a survival instinct, because we thrive in community and wilt in isolation. If you consider our ancestors – the ones who were chased by animals who saw them as dinner – you'll realize why we travel in packs. It's for physical protection. Translate that need to the 21st century and you'll find it transforms into *emotional* protection. We need to have people who understand us, so that we can face those who don't. We need people who worry about our safety, so that if the worst happens, they'll come to our rescue. We need people to lift us up, because modern life can kick us down more often than we'd like. We need people – and we are needed right back in return.

Connection is one of the greatest shields we have against mental illness. And yet, largely thanks to the stigma we've attached to depression and anxiety, when we feel low we choose isolation instead, because we think we're failing. This must change, because loneliness is more detrimental to our overall health than we realize. We must protect ourselves from it.

HOW DO WE BECOME SO LONELY?

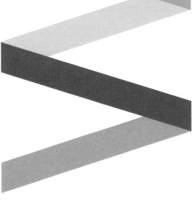

1

Something happens that makes a person feel isolated from their peers or community.

2

This leads to them feeling down about themselves and/or their life.

3

Feeling bad makes them withdraw even more, increasing their feelings of isolation.

4

Further withdrawal and negative thoughts lead to despair.

5

This can lead to depression and make the person hard to reach both physically and emotionally.

THE LONELINESS EPIDEMIC

We've all felt lonely at some point in our lives, if only fleetingly. Maybe we moved to a place where we didn't know anyone, or found ourselves in a situation where we were emotionally disconnected from those people we did know.

Loneliness is defined as often or always feeling lonely and it's having a big impact on our mental and physical health. It usually results when there's a mismatch between the quality and quantity of relationships that we have and those that we want. Luckily for most, these feelings pass, but more and more people (particularly Gen Zs) are experiencing what's known as chronic loneliness, that is to say, loneliness that is sustained for long periods of time. Things have become so bad that the World Health Organization (WHO) has acknowledged that we're living through an epidemic of loneliness.

It is clear to me that there are two forms of loneliness. Firstly, social loneliness is feeling a lack of belonging, companionship and/or membership of a community. Secondly, emotional loneliness is the lack of someone to turn to for advice or guidance, such as a parent, guardian or teacher. Neither type is good for our health.

People with diagnosed mental illness are more likely to be lonely, and lonely people are more likely to develop mental illness. A UK Office for National Statistics (ONS) report from 2021 found that rates of depression in adults were running at 21 per cent, a level that had doubled in two years. The ONS also reported that 3.7m over-16s experienced chronic loneliness, which is one in every 14 people.[5]

And loneliness does not just affect our mental wellbeing. It can wreak as much havoc on us physically, in the form of chronic diseases such as diabetes and high blood pressure. Research carried out by the Campaign to End Loneliness found that long-term loneliness can be worse for someone's health than obesity, even as bad for us as smoking 15 cigarettes a day.[6]

Just think about that for a minute!

Being lonely can be the driver for higher blood pressure, BMI, cholesterol, levels of the stress hormone cortisol and, ultimately, risk of early death. There are strong links between loneliness and poverty, unemployment and being shut out of normal society. Loneliness can lead to a lack of self-esteem or purpose, to depression and thoughts of ending one's life. All of which affect productivity, leading to issues with all sorts of things, including the ability to work effectively. And the saddest statistic of all is that lonely people are 50 per cent more likely to die than those with a good social network. So, clearly, we've got to get serious about how we connect.

You have to be honest
about four things:
what you want;
what you need;
what you feel;
who you are.

LIFESTYLE LOSSES

You can be surrounded by people, yet still feel alone. Even with the millions of followers I have on my socials, there are times when I feel lonely. If you took away my work, I'd say I'm probably a prime candidate for feeling lonely and isolated. And to be honest, if I'm not proactive, I do.

In the last five years, my social life has changed dramatically. Of course, that happens when you move from your 20s to your 30s, but I don't think we talk about it enough. Those transitions aren't always as easy as we'd expect, and they happen just as we start to build our lives and settle into our adulthood.

Everyone's pace in life is different, as are their choices, so when my friendship group started to up sticks, move out of London and start building families of their own, it did leave me feeling lonelier than ever before. I feel as if I've lost 80 per cent of my friendship group. I have four friends left in London – four very good friends, but only four nonetheless – and even then it can feel like a struggle to see them at times.

If I don't consciously plan how I'm going to spend my free time – and I'm guilty of dropping the ball on this a lot – then I will likely spend the weekend alone. That's not always a bad thing, but I'm aware enough now to know that I need social and emotional connection with my friends on a regular basis. They add immense value to my life, they're the people who know me better than anyone else. They matter.

When I do have a free weekend now, in which I have no plans to meet people, I'll make sure to get out for as many walks with the dog as possible. Being out and about means seeing people, whether we talk or not. The odd smile or nod can really chase away any hints of loneliness. We are all looking for connection, we just have to try to be proactive about it.

NOT ALL SOLITUDE IS LONELY

When I'm talking about loneliness, I'm talking about isolation and disconnection. That differs greatly from time to ourselves, which we often savour. People can quite happily spend time alone doing something they enjoy, or getting chores done, or even just being in the moment. There's nothing wrong with that – it can be nourishing – and it should be encouraged. But being contentedly alone seems to be something of a lost art and, due to the hyper-connected nature of modern living, solitude these days is equated with loneliness. We have so much connectivity with the online space that if we log off, even for a moment, we don't know what to do with ourselves. It's important that we give ourselves space and time to just *be*.

In the recent pandemic years, when we were forced to spend more time at home than ever before, I had to learn to enjoy my own company and be happy sitting at home with myself. It wasn't easy, but rather than feeling alone, or that I needed to be doing something, I learned to enjoy being present and practiced mindfulness daily (read more about that on page 156). I found quietening my mind and being with my thoughts a reflective process and quite beneficial. I found that even though I couldn't connect with others, I had connected with myself. And that's not loneliness, that's empowering.

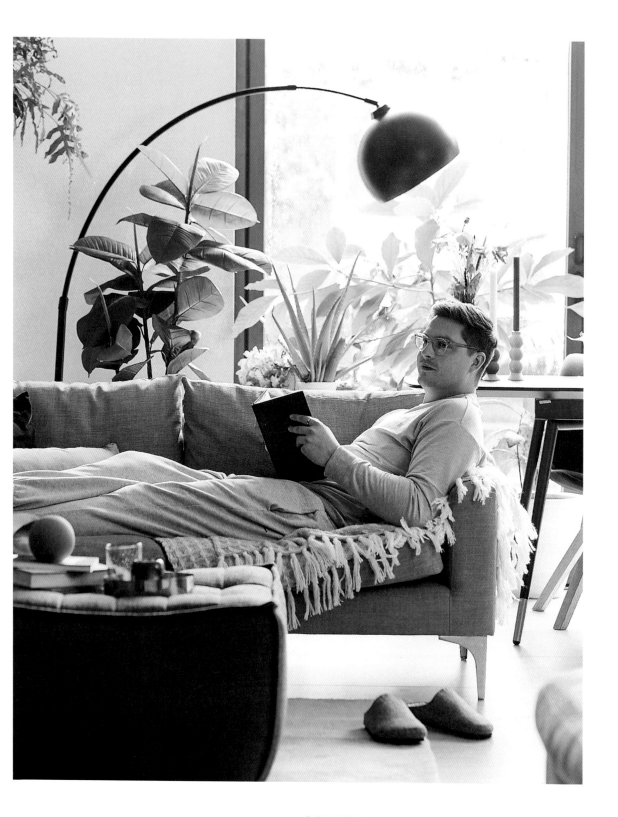

ACKNOWLEDGE THE DISCONNECT

We've all heard the trope that we are the most connected human beings in history. That social media has made our lives easier, more interactive and widened our friendship groups. And while, yes, those things are true in one respect, they don't give us the whole picture.

The reality is that when we use social media for hours of every day, we feel incredibly *disconnected* – oh, the irony! The constant social media attention thief creates an 'us and them' scenario, in which we spend more time wondering what other people are up to when they're not there than we do enjoying our own lives.

The only way we can combat loneliness is to acknowledge the disconnect we have in our lives. And if social media is causing you to feel isolated and lonely, then it's important to challenge your own narrative about using it. One of the most important lessons here is not necessarily in making the change, but in acknowledging that the problem might lie in the very device you think is helping you. Have a think about it, then make plans to shift things for yourself.

One of the most important ways to strengthen your mental health is to ensure that you are as connected to an in-person community (whether that be friends, family or neighbours) as possible. Research by Stanford University in the US found that social connection has the opposite effect on our physical health than loneliness does. Connection leads to a 50 per cent increased chance of longevity; strengthens your immune system; helps you recover from disease faster; even lengthens your life. On top of that, it is proven to reduce levels of anxiety and depression and people who feel connected to peers are shown to have higher self-esteem, greater empathy and are more trusting and cooperative.[7] Who wouldn't want all of that?

So, instead of using loneliness as another stick to beat yourself with, use it as a warning sign that you need more connection. Sometimes I think we forget as adults that our childhood lives were planned by our parents to give us all the connections we needed at a young age. But when we step out into adulthood, we often don't realize we need to take up the responsibility for doing that in our own lives. We need to organise 'play dates' with peers, take ourselves to 'after school' activities, sign up to 'summer camps'. We can – and should – do all these things for our adult selves.

At any point,
someone can come
along and change
your entire life.
That person is you.

SPREAD KINDNESS LIKE CONFETTI

On the most basic level, human beings crave connection – we simply can't function properly without it. We need to learn how important our interactions with others are, whether we know that person or not, rather than just taking those encounters for granted. We have the power to make the loneliness epidemic a thing of the past and to move forward to a kinder, more considerate society, without leaving anybody behind.

On an individual level, to increase our connection with the world, we need to make being kind a priority. It's the little gestures that matter most. If you catch someone's eye in the street, smile at them or say 'good morning', because you don't know how that might affect their day. They may not give it a second thought, but it may also give them a lift, especially if they're having a hard time. And let's not forget what that interaction is doing for your own mental health.

Every little bit of social interaction we experience throughout the day builds up our connection bank. I'm not talking about catching up with a good friend over coffee or having a long chat on the phone with a family member, although these are obviously really important and fulfilling.

What I'm referring to are those little interactions – they're called micro-connections – that we all have daily and that may go unnoticed.

Whether it be saying 'hello' to a stranger you see while out walking the dog, or exchanging a couple of words with a supermarket cashier, all these micro-connections add up to a sense of belonging and community. It's easy to underestimate the power of these micro-connections, but they're essential for stopping our disconnection from growing.

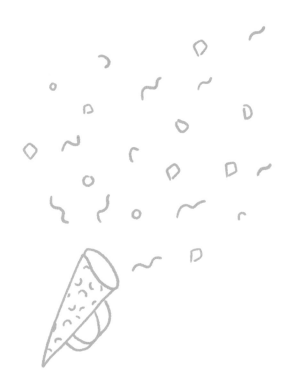

VOLUNTEER

Gen Zs and Millennials are not the only ones affected by loneliness these days. In 2019, four out of ten doctors reported regularly seeing elderly patients who were lonely and needed human attention, rather than requiring treatment for any medical condition.[8] I think we can confidently say that figure is now higher.

Even when I was working in emergency care, it was very common for an elderly person to come in with non-specific symptoms only to find, when you got to the bottom of it, that the reason they were there was because they felt very alone. They hadn't seen or even spoken to anyone for ages and felt distressed because of it. Emergency departments can be frenetic places at the best of times and you only want to visit one if you really *have* to. Seeing someone come in because they don't have anyone to turn to really stops you in your tracks.

That's why I recommend linking our generation with theirs through volunteering, meeting each group's need for connection. Offering your time to a local charity on a weekly basis is one of the easiest ways to combat loneliness. You get to interact with others and do some good for your community at the same time. Why not try working with a charity such as Age UK, which organizes social activities and befriending services for older people who are stuck at home? Or why not try a local food bank? A banker friend of mine volunteers at a food bank and finds it the most rewarding thing he's ever done. Try it for yourself. I can guarantee you'll learn, grow and have a lot of laughs.

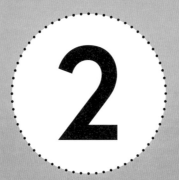

SLEEP WILL SAVE YOU

Your body needs rest, despite
what your work schedule suggests.
Use sleep to boost your brainpower
and watch your mood lift.

Sleep is the scaffolding of achievement. It is right up there with nutrition and exercise when it comes to good health, even more so when it comes to good mental health. Yet we're getting less sleep than ever. According to The Sleep Charity, almost three-quarters of us fail to get the minimum recommendation of seven hours of sleep each night. One-third of us sleep so poorly most nights that our energy levels and mood are constantly low. Around one-third of us feel our health, work and relationships are suffering.[9]

The same report found that 30–40 per cent of adults go through a period of chronic, debilitating sleeplessness, while 10 per cent experience chronic insomnia, a long-term inability to sleep.

Suffice it to say, we are facing a poor-sleep crisis that is undermining our health. For something so important to our wellbeing, it's often low down on the list of our health priorities. The bottom line is, we are not sleeping well, and it's having a devastating effect on our ability to live happy and successful lives.

WHAT SLEEP DOES TO OUR BRAINS

Someone who's had a profound impact on my attitude to sleep is Professor Matthew Walker. He's a neuroscientist, founder of the Center for Human Sleep Science at UC Berkeley in the US and author of *Why We Sleep*. Professor Walker is the heavyweight champion of getting seven-plus hours of shut-eye a night and what he doesn't know about sleep isn't worth knowing. His take on the importance of sleep is as straightforward as it is irrefutable. 'Sleep isn't an optional lifestyle luxury,' he says. 'Sleep is a non-negotiable biological necessity. It is your life support system.'

The main misconception people have about sleep – and before I became familiar with Professor Walker's work, I was guilty of this, too – is that it is a passive process. We think of sleep as downtime, as rest, as if our bodies simply shut down and don't do anything… except keep breathing, of course! But that couldn't be further from the truth. While we sleep, our bodies undertake a series of functions that impact every single biological process, affecting our cardiovascular, metabolic and mental health.

Sleep is a restorative process for both body and mind. There is not an organ in the body that doesn't benefit. But as far as your brain function is concerned, getting decent shut-eye enhances cognition, processing, memory, logic, learning and decision making. If you fail to get enough sleep, all that is going to suffer.

Studies have shown that less than seven hours of sleep causes measurable impairment in both our brains and our bodies. They also show that a lack of sleep can result in a 40 per cent learning deficit, which means we have a significantly lower capacity to retain new information when we are sleep deprived. Plus, the effect of 17 hours without sleep on our alertness and wakefulness is equivalent to the effects of a blood alcohol concentration of 0.05 per cent – not far off the UK legal limit for driving. (And after 24 hours without sleep, it goes up to 0.1 per cent, which is *over* the UK legal limit for driving.) There are so many things we wouldn't do when drunk and we shouldn't do them when we're sleep deprived either!

OPTIMUM SLEEP CYCLES

Each of these cycles has five stages: drowsiness, light sleep, two stages of deep sleep, Rapid Eye Movement (REM) sleep.

- ○ awake
- ● drowsiness
- ● REM
- ○ light sleep
- ● deep sleep stage 1
- ● deep sleep stage 2

You wake up briefly between most cycles, but don't tend to remember.

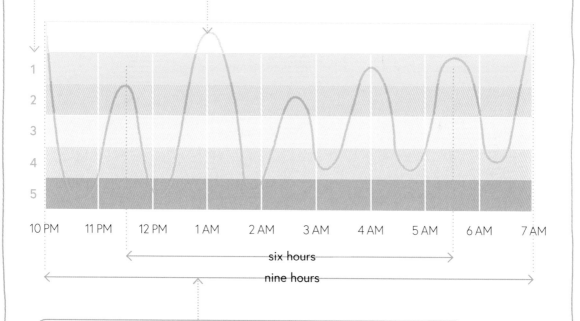

On average, we clock between six and nine hours of sleep at night, in four or five separate cycles, each lasting roughly ninety minutes.

A healthy adult's sleep comprises around 25 per cent deep sleep, 50 per cent light sleep and 25 per cent REM.

WHAT GOES ON WHILE WE SLEEP?

Sleep scientists break a night's sleep down into physiological stages. Far from being a passive state, there are plenty of things going on during our different stages of sleep.

Rapid Eye Movement (REM) sleep – in which we do most of our dreaming – provides a form of overnight therapy and helps us to process recent events and evaluate them subconsciously. You can think of dream sleep as mental first aid. It really can remove the emotional sting from troubling experiences, so who wouldn't want to stock up on it?

What's more, the two stages of deep sleep can help to reduce anxiety. The deeper we sleep, the greater the reduction, as it rewires our frontal lobe as well as the brain centres that trigger anxiety. Anxiety builds while we're awake, so without sleep to reduce it, the more anxious we feel.

There are physiological benefits to sleep as well. When we sleep, our brain cleans itself by flushing out the toxic proteins that are by-products of waking neural activity. This process – known as autophagy – removes dead blood cells and other waste products, improving the brain's functionality while promoting the growth of new cells. It's like having someone come in and give our brain a deep clean while we're snoring.

Another downside to skimping on pillow time is feeling emotionally fragile and struggling with situations that wouldn't normally cause us any problems. If that sounds familiar, it's because lack of sleep really affects our waking time. Sleep deprivation causes the rational, decision-making part of our brain – called the prefrontal cortex – to power down. So normal situations, that we usually cope with well, can feel overwhelming. The emotional part of our brain, called the amygdala, becomes super-sensitive... and so can we. We might feel more tearful, nervous or short-tempered.

SLEEP AND MENTAL IMBALANCE

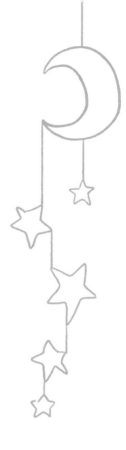

By now, you'll understand how important sleep is for good mental health. As Professor Walker points out, there is no major psychiatric condition in which good sleep is normal. Issues such as depression, anxiety and PTSD (see pages 197–199) all go hand-in-hand with sleep problems.

It was always thought that mental illness disrupted sleep, but Professor Walker indicates that this isn't always the case. Healthy people can experience neurological patterns similar to mental illness simply by having their sleep disrupted or blocked. That's because many of the regions of the brain involved in regulating sleep and and our circadian rhythms are the same as those impacted by mental illness. Sleep and mental imbalance are, therefore, intrinsically linked.

On the plus side, what that means is that improving sleep quantity, quality and regularity can help with mental illness and even *reverse* some of the symptoms.[10] For example, when it comes to mental wellness, night owls definitely come off worse than early birds... and not just in the worm-catching stakes. A recent study found that shifting sleep and waking up times earlier by just one hour may reduce the risk of developing depression by 23 per cent.[11]

Researchers found that those who tended to stay up late, and rise later, could benefit by going to bed just an hour earlier, even if the actual time spent asleep was the same. The reasons for the improvement in mental health included longer exposure to daylight, the hormonal benefits of which can boost mood. Then there's simply being awake when most other people are, helping potential sufferers of depression feel better connected and not excluded – something late risers might unwittingly feel.

Ensuring we go through all the stages of sleep – particularly REM and the two stages of deep sleep – means that our brains are being looked after in the way they're designed to be. Sleep is by far the best, and most natural, form of therapy.

TIPS FOR A GREAT NIGHT'S SLEEP

You spend more time in bed than anywhere else, so make sure your mattress, pillow and bedlinen are of good quality and encourage calm. There's nothing worse than scratchy sheets or a lumpy pillow: don't do it to yourself.

Stop using light-activated devices two hours before bedtime. Your eyes need to adjust each time you check that phone screen and this will keep you awake for longer.

If you struggle with intrusive thoughts when you hit the hay, keep a journal beside your bed. Empty your worries out on to a page and write down everything that's bothering you before your head touches the pillow.

Keep intense exercise for early in the day and avoid it within three hours of bedtime. You want your heart and body to be ebbing towards relaxation, which a high-intensity workout will destroy.

Avoid alcohol for a deep night's sleep. You may think it helps you to drop off, but it's actually robbing you of the most beneficial stages of sleep.

Expose yourself to daylight within an hour of waking in the morning. Getting natural light, when the season permits it, syncs you with your circadian rhythms.

Keep your bedroom cool and dark. The temperature sweet spot is 15–19°C (59–66°F).

Clean up your caffeine intake. Stop drinking it after 2pm.

PRACTICING WHAT I PREACH

Just a few years back, I believed that time in bed was wasted time, so I'd try to exist on as little sleep as possible. I'm now much more aware of how important sleep is and I'm very protective of it.

Nowadays, I go to bed at about 10pm and try to be asleep by 10:30pm. My alarm is set for 7am and I know that I need seven hours minimum a night, so I take into account how long it takes me both to fall asleep and to wake up in the morning, as well as the possibility that I might wake in the night. What this means is that I now feel really refreshed and restored when I wake; it has made a massive difference for me.

I've set some sleep hygiene rules for myself. Unless I've got a long drive ahead of me, I've started to stay away from caffeine after midday, as I find that really helps to keep my sleep patterns regular. If I have time, I'll have a nice warm, scented bath just before bed to unwind. When it comes to my phone, once I set the alarm for waking, I put it down and won't touch it again until the next morning. And then just as I'm getting into bed, I'll play some soothing piano-based music, which I find really calming – I can just drift away with it. I'll also take this music with me if I'm staying away from home, because it's important to have a consistent bedtime routine.

I view my bedroom differently too. I used to have an open-plan apartment, which looked cool but meant I was woken up by the fridge ticking over in the night. But now my bedroom is completely geared towards sleep. I invested in a comfortable mattress, installed a really thick blackout curtain and now keep the temperature constant. It's not a busy room: there's not much in it, no blue lights or TV, just a few plants. It's basically a sleep haven!

All of this has come together and I now sleep a lot better and definitely feel the benefit. During the day I'm better focused, more attentive and generally happier and so is everyone around me! I'm more present in my days and I get more out of them – not always in terms of productivity necessarily, but definitely in terms of enjoyment.

If I had to choose only one thing that I think can make the most difference to the most people, it would be getting the right amount of good-quality sleep. It's quite literally the best thing we can do for ourselves.

SLEEP FOR SUCCESS

People rarely talk about sleep and, if they do, you don't hear many people boasting about what a great sleeper they are. It's just not celebrated in the same way other health-supporting activities are. In fact, it's kind of the opposite, and I'd like to change that.

'Sleep is for wimps,' 'I'm too busy to sleep,' or 'I'll sleep when I'm dead,' are mantras that I've heard both from friends and colleagues, as well as on TV. The latter is a phrase I particularly dislike. Not only because it smacks of a certain type of toxic productivity, but also because, if anything is going to cut short our mortality, it's lack of sleep.

The idea that to be successful we need to work long hours, forgo downtime and stay up late is still with us. But missing out on sleep in order to work harder is among the greatest lies we've been told. In fact, it's completely counterproductive.

One thing that we're not really acknowledging is that long hours don't just mean those spent at the office or over a desk. Modern life seems expect us to be always 'on call', whether we work as doctors or not. It seems many industries have leaned into the bad habits of sending emails at 2am, expecting immediate responses no matter what the time, or sending voice notes when a thought occurs rather than noting it down and delivering it at an appropriate moment. If we're not careful with who can reach us and when, we can be open for business 24/7. We have to set boundaries for ourselves and hope that others will follow.

We need to reframe the idea of what hard work is. If we're not rested, we're less effective and therefore have to work harder to compensate for that. Being able to do our jobs more effectively because we've had enough sleep is a far better thing than doing them badly for longer hours. The mantra 'work smarter, not harder' has been around for a while and it is *so* true. It just stands to reason: well-rested and motivated workers are far more productive than fatigued people.

Thankfully, the tide seems to be turning. When author Arianna Huffington was Editor-in-Chief at *The Huffington Post*, she used to survive on three to four hours of sleep a night. Until, one day, she collapsed and was diagnosed with exhaustion. It was a turning point and, in her book *The Sleep Revolution*, she tells us how changing her sleep habits revolutionized her life. She makes a strong case for good sleep being of the utmost importance to our mental, emotional and physical health.

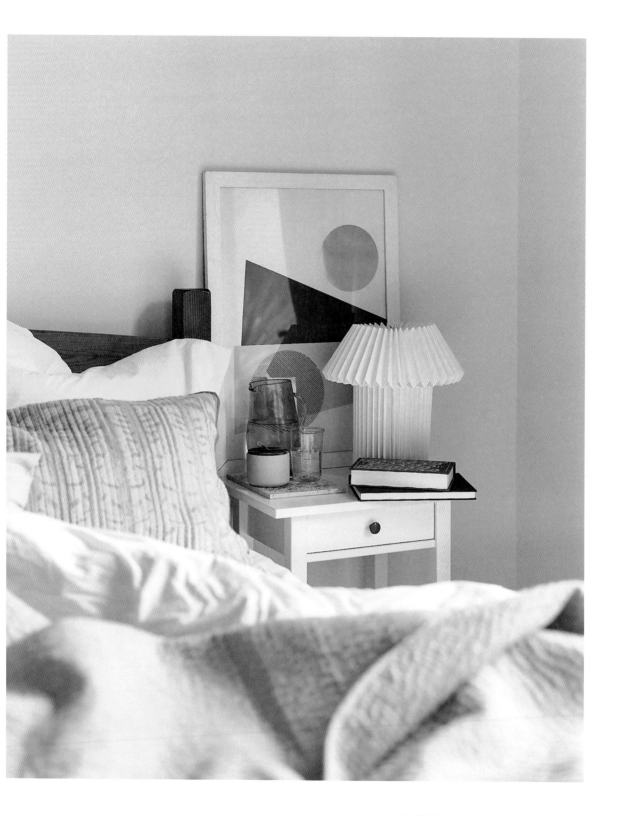

You are way more
capable than you
could ever imagine.

CARRY OUT A SLEEP AUDIT

Sleep is a powerful performance enhancer, but I appreciate not all of us have the luxury of increasing how much of it we get. New parents, carers and shift workers all have valid reasons for not being able to get the amount of sleep I've talked about in this chapter! As always, my aim here isn't to sleep-shame anyone or to cause anxiety, so if changing your sleep habits isn't something you can do right now, don't worry. You're now armed with all the knowledge you need to make the change whenever you can.

The small lifestyle tweaks really do count the most. Here are some questions to get you started with an audit of your sleeping status:

- ☐ **Could I stop drinking caffeine earlier in the day?**

- ☐ **Do I need that nightcap?**

- ☐ **Can I go screen-free for at least two hours before bedtime?**

- ☐ **Could I swap my smartphone/TV/laptop/games console for a warm bath and a good book in bed?**

- ☐ **Is my bedroom a calm, clutter-free place that feels relaxing?**

- ☐ **Is my bedroom as quiet, cool, dark and comfortable as I can make it?**

- ☐ **Do I have a plan for if I can't sleep, or if I wake in the night?**

For the last question, my advice – gleaned from many a sleep expert – is to get up if you're awake for more than a few minutes. Don't lie there ruminating. Go and make yourself herbal tea or warm milk. Head to another room and do something that isn't too stimulating – read a book or magazine or listen to gentle music – as opposed to firing up any sort of screen. Then, when you start to feel sleepy, head back to bed, trying not to watch the clock.

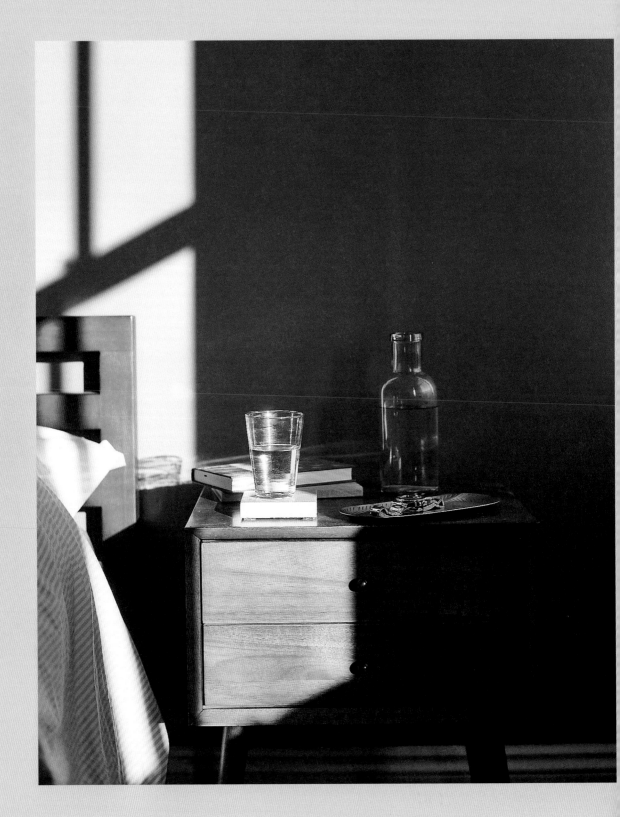

REMOVE DEVICES

The one thing you could do to help you sleep better *tonight* is to find a new spot for your devices to charge. If your current MO sees you charge your phone beside your bed, or keep it there because you need it as an alarm in the morning, then I'd suggest finding it a new bedtime home. Doing so will remove the temptation to check the time during the night, when the phone's bright light will wake you up from your calm state. It will also mean that notification sounds don't disrupt your sleep. You could switch on the Do Not Disturb function, but overall I think it's best to remove the device from the room entirely. Find yourself an alarm clock, or leave your phone just outside the bedroom door so you can still hear its alarm, thus forcing you up out of bed without hitting the snooze button too many times. Win-win!

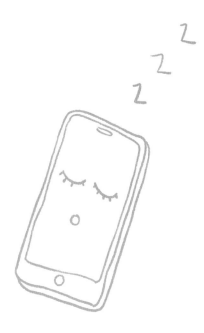

BOUNDARIES ARE BEAUTIFUL

Having boundaries is key to mental fitness and lots of us need to reclaim our lives from the expectations of a society that never says 'no'.

Be honest with yourself: how many times have you said 'yes' to something, then immediately regretted it? Social events, overtime, helping people out… at some point we've all agreed to do something or go somewhere when we know, deep down, we really didn't want to. Why don't we speak up for our own boundaries?

There are many reasons why we feel uncomfortable saying 'no', but if we could manage it just a little more often, the benefits for our free time and stress levels would be huge.

As with many issues, the origins to our 'no' resistance can be found in childhood: perhaps we said 'yes' to keep our parents happy and that's turned us into people-pleasers. Now, as adults, it's the social uncertainty of what kind of response a 'no' will elicit that makes us reluctant to turn people down. Will we upset them, make them angry, will they lose respect for us? Sometimes the thought of the potential reaction to a 'no' makes it seem simpler to just say 'yes'.

THE SWAY OF IMPULSE

Social conditioning aside, there is a physiological reason why saying 'yes' is, initially at least, preferable to saying 'no'. All our responses are framed by our impulses and different parts of our brain are more impulsive than others. Unfortunately for us, it's the impulsive parts that have most sway over our initial responses.

The psychologist Steve Peters, author of *The Chimp Paradox*, has a great analogy for explaining this. Professor Peters, who's best known for his work with the UK Olympic cyclists Victoria Pendleton and Sir Bradley Wiggins, refers to the impulsive part of our brain – the limbic system – as our inner chimp. It's the chimp who is impulsive, makes rash decisions and is involved in those instantaneous fight-or-flight responses that used to keep us safe from sabre-toothed tigers back when we were cave dwellers.

Obviously, since then, we've evolved a bit and developed a more measured side to our brains.

This is known as the prefrontal cortex and houses our sensible, rational side. The trouble is that first, the inner chimp is the more powerful of the two, and second, that new information tends to go by the chimp before it reaches the prefrontal cortex. Which is why we make rash decisions that we subsequently regret.

Professor Peters worked with British Cycling to explore the use of tools to manage the inner chimp, to ensure athletes didn't make rash decisions while competing. They learned to unleash their inner ape only when it would benefit their performance.

That said, humans are hardwired to say 'yes', and doing so immediately appeases the reward centres of our brains. We get an immediate dopamine response and feel elated, but that can be followed by anxiety and, sometimes, resentment. It's always worth taking your time when making decisions, so you can manage the inner chimp and answer with your prefrontal cortex.

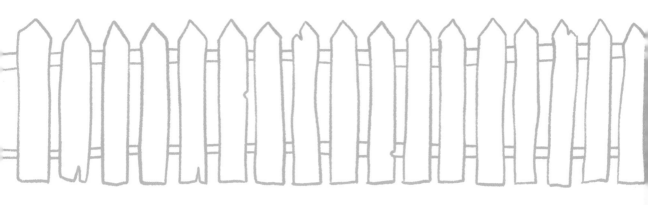

YOU'RE ONLY HURTING YOURSELF

You've said 'yes' to something you either don't want or don't really have the capacity to do. Maybe it's an extra shift at work, babysitting your nieces, or a weekend away for a friend's birthday. You're dreading it, you suffer during it because you're not as engaged as you need to be, then afterwards you're tired and annoyed because you now don't have the energy to do something you actually want to do. It's almost painful.

In his book *The Power of No*, entrepreneur James Altucher says, 'When you say yes to something you don't want to, here is the result: you hate what you are doing, you resent the person who asked you, and you hurt yourself.'

Unfortunately, people who say 'yes' to everything end up doing a lot of things averagely, rather than doing a few things amazingly. It's something I can identify with: in the past, I've definitely said 'yes' to too many things. But as demands on my time have increased, I've learned how to keep that impulse in check and have felt much happier and more accomplished for it. For me, the power of saying 'no' has made me more productive. 'No' allows me to say 'yes' to things I want to do, then to do them well.

There really is a power to saying 'no'. You're enforcing your boundaries and looking after yourself. Being sensitive predisposes us to worry about other people's opinions and pushes us to say 'yes'. But we can't control how others interpret our 'no'. If they're going to get upset, then they're going to get upset. At first it will be hard, but it does get easier. And, eventually, people will respect you for it.

These days, I say 'no' a lot of more, yet I'm still busy. It's tough, because the people-pleaser in me wants to say 'yes' all the time. I don't like letting people down, yet I'm hyper-aware that I have to make the best account of myself possible whenever I've agreed to something. If I'm being asked to do anything to which I can't give my total focus, then I'm not going to be doing my best.

DO YOU HAVE CAPACITY?

Think about this scenario: you're invited by three different groups of friends to play tennis, basketball or football. You could do all three, but that would mean holding back on the first two, so by the time you get to the third you won't be too tired to play. Or you could do two of the sports and only partially commit to each. Or you could choose just one and give it 100 per cent. Which do you feel more comfortable with? For me, it's giving something my full focus, so I keep that in mind when I have to say 'no' to something.

Lining the options up like this is a great way to figure out if you have the capacity for something that is asked of you. Consider if something is a 'need to do', such as a work project, or a 'want to do', such as meeting up with friends. If you say 'yes' to one, will that mean you have the energy to commit to the other? And if the answer is 'no', then say it. It's about figuring out your priorities and saying 'no' to everything that isn't on the list.

'NO' IS A COMPLETE SENTENCE

If you're having trouble locating your inner 'no', then get a little bit angry. Not with the person asking you to do something, but with all the time you've wasted in the past when you said 'yes' to something you didn't want to do. How many social occasions have you attended that you wished you hadn't? How many boring meetings have you found yourself in when there was no reason for you to be there? And it's not just time, but money too. Going out is expensive and that's galling when you didn't want to be there in the first place.

Once you've found your 'no', focus on what saying it more often will give you. Think of the extra time, the extra money, the capacity to do the things you want – or are better placed – to do well.

Imbue the word 'no' with the positives usually associated with saying 'yes'.

Then think about situations about which you wished you'd said 'no' in the past and imagine what it would have been like if you *had* said it then. Write them down if it helps. As my parents used to ask me, 'What's the worst that could have happened?' Would someone have been upset with you? Angry? Sad? Disappointed? Would the positives of saying 'no' in such situations have outweighed the negatives of saying 'yes'?

Never judge someone's story by the chapter you walked in on.

THE NOTHING OF 'NO'

Saying 'no' allows you to say 'yes' to things that are important to you, but it also gives you time to do … nothing. And I mean really do nothing. With all our busy-ness and devices and social media platforms, we have forgotten how to just be. To be still. To be bored. If time is our most valuable currency, then we're currently handing it over to our employers and tech companies, when perhaps we should be keeping a little for ourselves.

Even at work, giving your brain a break can pay dividends for your creativity. Having nothing to do has been scientifically proven to be beneficial for creative thinking, because when our brains are relaxed our prefrontal cortex – the bit of the brain that deals with attention, memory and planning – goes on autopilot and allows our minds to wander. Work futurist Dominic Price suggests that employers should allow their workers some scheduled boredom time every week, for exactly this reason. Price calls this the 'anti-power hour' and thinks it could revolutionize how we approach creativity in the workplace.[12]

You're not too
sensitive and you're
not overreacting.
If it hurts you,
it hurts.

THE CULT OF BUSY-NESS

We've all been there. You're catching up with a friend and inevitably the conversation comes around to work. 'How's it going?' you ask. 'Oh, really busy,' comes the answer, normally swiftly followed by, 'But mustn't complain.' I've said it myself many times and although it may have been true (I was a junior doctor after all), telling people that you're 'super-busy' is still – at the very least – a humblebrag, if not an outright boast. But why has being busy become such a badge of honour?

It doesn't just apply to work. On social media, being super-productive has become a status symbol. The actor Mark Wahlberg once shared his daily routine on Instagram. It included getting up at 2:30am, multiple workouts and a 7:30pm bedtime. It was immediately parodied, but it did highlight how simply showing people how busy you are had become a productivity flex, rather than something to inspire others. The idea of achieving everything you want to do while not having any downtime creates a false goal – it is an illusion – and results in unhealthy comparisons. It's certainly not something I'd recommend.

When I was a junior doctor, many of the consultants used to regale us with stories of how, in the past, they would work 120 hours a week. It was intimidating to hear that, but there was also an unspoken suggestion that we were failing if we weren't doing such insane hours. I came to realize that such expectations were unrealistic and unhealthy. Having to work 120 hours a week is not something to brag about… and something is going very wrong in the workplace if you are.

The stereotype that junior doctors work very long hours definitely has a basis in reality. I still shudder when I think of the 12-days-in-a-row shifts we used to have to work. But I'd be lying if I said there wasn't a small part of me that felt proud of being so busy and frantic. I'd come off one of those shifts on a high (probably due to exhaustion), then we'd all go to the pub, get drunk and feel awful the next day. But I think that's where the badge-of-honour stuff comes from: we were proud that we got through it. Looking back, I can now appreciate that I ate terribly for those 12 days, I didn't go to the gym and I was mentally and physically exhausted. Rather than relaxing, I had a night out, which exacerbated things further. I'd end up sleeping all weekend and then go into work on Monday feeling just as tired. It was an unsustainable and unhealthy way to live.

Toxic productivity like that leads to burnout, because such ridiculous standards of 'achievement' are impossible to maintain. The irony is that it actually makes us less productive. But most of all, these humblebrags and busy-ness flexes tell us that, as a society, we really don't know how to say 'no'.

FIND YOUR ANCHOR PHRASE

Not ready to deploy your 'no' just yet? Still think your inner chimp
is going to vault over your prefrontal cortex and blurt out 'yes'?
Then buy yourself some time with what's known as an anchor phrase.
It's basically a stalling tactic that can give you a bit of headspace to sort
out your response. This is something I use a lot, not only because it gives
me time to think about what I want, but also to check my schedule.
When I'm asked to make a decision that's not an obvious 'yes',
I say, 'Ask me again tomorrow.'

It may sound ridiculously simple, but it is an incredibly effective
system and one that stops me from making unrealistic commitments.
It pays to choose an anchor phrase, learn it and get used to saying it,
so that you can employ it any time you find yourself in an uncomfortable
situation. Once you've given yourself that space, you can formulate
a response that considers who is doing the asking and their likely reaction.
You can use mine, or try out: 'Let me get back to you on that,' 'Let me check
my schedule,' 'Can I sleep on that?' 'I've got a feeling
I'm booked up that day, but I'll let you know later.'

An anchor phrase is also good for preventing you from making a rash
decision if you're on the back foot emotionally. You should never make
a decision when you're reeling from a loss or a victory, because it's going to
influence you in some way. A decision that comes from a place of emotion
rather than calculation can often be one you regret.

YOU HAVE NOTHING TO APOLOGIZE FOR

There's a societal pressure to preface a refusal with a 'sorry' or 'I'm afraid', which suggests that you've done something wrong. Please don't do that. It's not rude to not be sorry for turning something down. We need to be a little less fearful about saying 'no'. Think of it as a transaction, in which your time is as valuable as that of others. If they have nothing worth investing your time in, then you shouldn't feel guilty about that. Be polite, of course, but don't say sorry. You have absolutely nothing to apologize for.

This is not to say that you should never say sorry. If you have actually done something wrong, if you've dropped the ball, or perhaps want to say 'no' now after saying 'yes' before, then you should say sorry. The overall message is to be kind, both to yourself and to others. If you use that rule of thumb, you'll find it easier to avoid apologizing for your boundaries.

This may all sound easier said than done, and it would be unrealistic of me to say it didn't take practice, because it can be a big perception shift for many of us. But establishing healthy boundaries, knowing your capacity – and feeling empowered enough to protect it – is so important for mental health and wellbeing.

Start with the small stuff at first: those after-work drinks and group invitations where your absence won't be so keenly felt. Then, once you've got the confidence, start saying 'no' to things that in the past have been more difficult to turn down. After a while, people will realize that you say 'yes' to the things that are important to you. They – and you – will know you'll be bringing your best self, whether that's to a social event, a work project or simply spending time with someone. Being present and attentive is a much more generous way to give your time to others than by doing it begrudgingly.

THE TOKEN APPROACH

When I find my energy being drawn away from those things to which I should be giving all my focus, I look at my life in terms of tokens.

Imagine that every day you have a certain number of tokens. Whether they're tokens of energy or time or emotional focus, they're a currency and you have a limited amount to spend. Once you've spent them, you have nothing left, so if you do continue to spend then you're borrowing from the next day's tokens, or even from the day after that. And if you carry on doing that, soon you'll be in a deficit in real terms. This is burnout. I find that this helps me think about two things: what I want to commit to every day, and to be mindful of the fact that there's only so much I can do in 24 hours. And it informs my decision-making when it comes to saying 'yes' or 'no'.

I recently used this strategy when deciding to give the biggest 'no' of my life to date. As my work is increasingly about campaigning and getting out and meeting people, I'm finding I've got fewer and fewer tokens to spend on clinical medicine. I believe my work in the mental health arena is part of my purpose: it's doing some real good in terms of helping young people navigate this strange time in which we find ourselves. But I can't be in two places at once, so there came a time when I had to make a decision. And that decision was to leave clinical medicine for the time being. It was a difficult 'no' to say, because I really enjoy working in emergency medicine and I love going back to my hospital in southeast London. I like the work and I feel I'm being useful there, but it just came to a point where I had to admit that I can't do everything. So I've paused my A&E work to focus full-time on mental health advocacy, including returning to university to study a master's degree in Public Mental Health. Who knows what the future will bring? But I know now that I can make hard decisions for the sake of my own health, while also following those opportunities that fill me with passion.

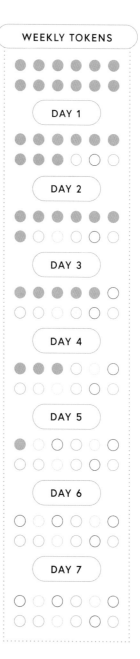

WEEKLY TOKENS

DAY 1

DAY 2

DAY 3

DAY 4

DAY 5

DAY 6

DAY 7

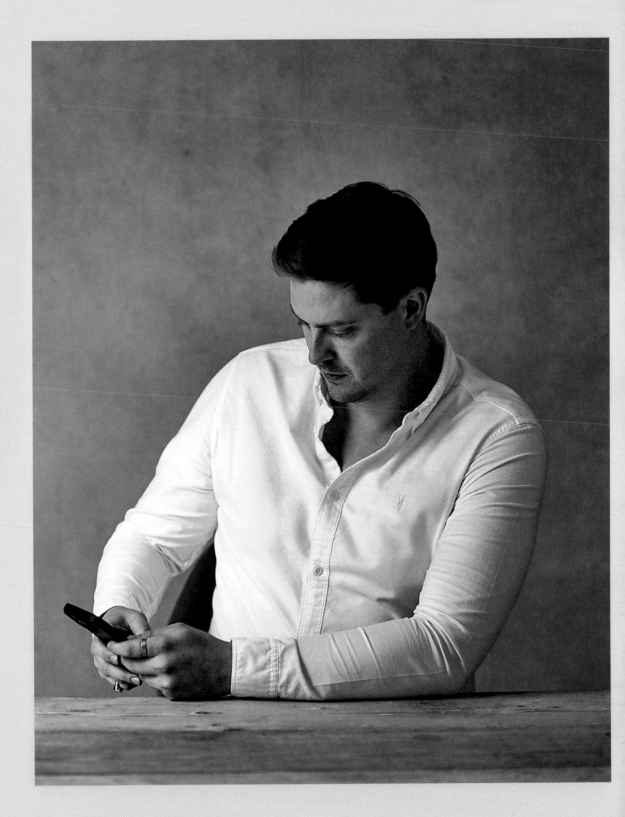

CONSIDER THE PAYOFF

Still struggling to locate your inner 'no'? Wondering where you'll find the confidence to turn things down? Then think about this: by constantly saying 'yes' to things that make you unhappy, you are literally wasting your life. Your time on this earth is limited; you won't get back any of it that is wasted on things you don't want to do.

How much of your life do you spend being happy and fulfilled? I'm not talking about being simply content, but completely at peace, engaged and inspired? Whether with other people or alone, this is how you should be spending the majority of your time. If you still enjoy the busy-ness flex, well, you can still be busy spending more time with friends and family, or use the extra capacity to start that project you've always talked about. Whatever you decide to do, it will benefit your own mental wellbeing.

NO TIME LIKE NOW

SAY 'NO'

Look at what you've got coming up in your calendar and find something you really don't want to do. Then write an email, send a text or make a phone call to remove it from your diary.

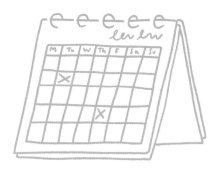

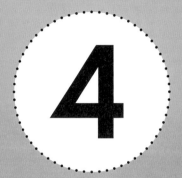

MISTAKES ARE
A MUST-HAVE

Never fear mistakes. The only way you will
ever learn is by making them. Learn how to
make them work for you, not against you.

Have you ever missed out on an opportunity because you were afraid of making mistakes or failing? Are there things you haven't done because you were worried about the consequences? Maybe you didn't apply for a job, or try out for a team, for fear of rejection. Perhaps you never put your hand up in class in case you gave the wrong answer. Or didn't go and speak to that person you'd been admiring, worried you'd be turned down.

If any of the above are familiar to you, then you've experienced a fear of failure. Don't worry, it's very common, so much so that in its extreme form it is even classed as a phobia. I fail every day. There, I've admitted it and I don't feel guilty or ashamed. And why should I? Failure is part of life and I believe you learn more from your failures than you do from your successes. Getting things wrong and making mistakes can be painful and it can be hard at first to see the positives. But looking back at my own experiences, I feel grateful for what I learned from them.

Fear of failing is part of human nature: it exists to keep us from harm. But, like an overprotective parent, it can stop us from achieving our potential and sabotage our chances of success, not to mention eroding our self-worth and making us unhappy.

It impacts everyone and anyone. The perception that a fear of failing affects only low achievers couldn't be further from the truth. A recent US study found that 90 per cent of all CEOs fear failure.[13] But you don't have to be the head of a big company with a lot on the line to feel anxious about making mistakes. It's all about context: even the smallest failure can have an impact. A failure may be objectively small, but to the person who has failed it can be huge.

What are we afraid of exactly? Top of the list is anxiety about what others may think of our failure, of being humiliated in front of our peers. Worrying about the opinions of others is unfortunately very common, and many people's whole identity is tied up with being accepted by societal groups. Failing in front of those groups – and a fear of rejection by them because of it – is very real. You would think, then, that such powerful anxiety would be based on prior experience, or at least a set of evidence proving that such a rejection will happen. Not so. It's usually the uncertainty surrounding what *might* happen when you fail that's more worrying to people than the failure itself.[14] And sadly, for increasing numbers of people, this 'what if' is stopping them from living full and fulfilling lives.

WHAT'S THE EFFECT ON OUR MENTAL HEALTH?

While I'm sure there are confident, secure people out there who may question whether fear of failure actually exists, I can assure them that it does. Taken to the extreme, it is a diagnosable condition recognized as a phobia: atychiphobia, an irrational and persistent fear of failing. Extreme or not, it affects all genders, young and old, rich and poor. Medically speaking, it can stop people enjoying life and their achievements, leaving them unfulfilled and prone to self-doubt and worry, which in turn can lead to anxiety, isolation and depression.

And all these things can have a negative impact on our mental health. Add to that the stigma attached to failure – the shame, the embarrassment, the guilt – which makes it hard to talk about, or to admit to, making mistakes.

Talking about failure is key to taking away its power. Fear of failure can only be a stress factor in our lives if we let it. But first we have to have a safe space in which we can discuss it. Only then can we have a say in how we respond.

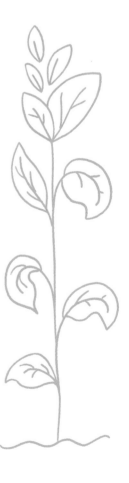

REFRAME FAILURE AS GROWTH

Thomas Edison, inventor of the lightbulb, is reported to have once said, 'I have not failed, I have found several thousand things that won't work.' I find that *such* an inspirational quote – despite the fact that Edison probably never actually said it! – because it sums up everything I believe about the importance of making mistakes. Errors are not about getting something wrong, they are a necessary step on the path to getting it right.

In her book *Mindset*, author Carol Dweck writes that mistakes are the best way to learn, and that a shift in mindset is all that is needed to reframe failure. She believes we either have a fixed mindset – in which we believe we already know everything we need to about a given subject and that no more learning can happen – or a growth mindset, in which we approach everything with the view that we can learn as we go; that we will always be learning and growing. She says that mindset change is about seeing things in a new way: 'When people change to a growth mindset, they change from a judge-and-be-judged framework to a learn-and-help-learn framework. Their commitment is to growth, and growth takes plenty of time, effort, and mutual support.'

The idea is that we don't show up as fully rounded experts in every field. Some of us can have particular talents, but even to allow those to bloom, we need to take action, try, fail… and try again. Dweck uses athletes as examples. These people are human beings, not wonderkids; it does us no favours to think of them as infallible. They make mistakes, just like the rest of us. And if anyone knows how to work their growth mindset, it's British Formula One champion Sir Lewis Hamilton. Until the 2021 season it would've been easy to think of his reign as a consistent rise, but it had a start-stop beginning. Hamilton won his first championship in 2008 when he was 23, but spent the next 6 years fighting to regain that title. He threw everything he could into the sport, he tried thousands of ways that didn't work, then eventually, in 2014, the hard work paid off and he won the second of his seven championships to date. He went on to win every year bar one: in the 2021 season, a controversial mid-race decision in the final race saw him lose out to Max Verstappen. Instead of playing the sore loser card, Hamilton complained through the right channels, accepted the decision, then put his head down to plan for the next season. That next season, 2022, saw some major engineering changes take effect and Hamilton started it off with frustration. But as with anyone who possess a growth mindset, he kept at it, trying and failing week-on-week, until things started to improve. He climbed the rankings and made the most of the challenge by learning, even after 15 years at the top of the sport. We can all learn from Hamilton, as well as from other athletes who spend hours honing their craft. They are not superhuman. They did not wake up that good. They put the hours in. And the only way they got to be as good as they are is by failing again and again. If it's good enough for Lewis Hamilton, it's good enough for me!

You aren't a failure
for having bad days.
You aren't a burden
for having bad days.
You aren't a bad person
for having bad days.

HARMFUL HASHTAGS

Whether consciously or not, social media and its obsession with celebrating success – #livingmybestlife – puts added pressure on users, particularly Gen Z who spend the most time on those platforms. On Instagram, for example, the two biggest anxiety-inducing pressures are the presentation of perfection and of high productivity. This creates a sense of 'never enoughness': those highs of perfection and productivity are just too far up to reach. And that's because they aren't real, they don't show the whole picture.

I used to be particularly susceptible to the high productivity pressure, as I hated the idea that I was not maximizing my productivity each day. When I saw others doing more than me, I felt lazy and unproductive. Thankfully, over the past couple of years, I've separated myself from that. But it is something I've seen time and time again and it's beginning to be recognized as a form of 'toxic positivity'.

For my part, I try to strike a balance between putting positive, inspirational posts on social media and ones that just tell it like it is. I think it's important to show a well-rounded view of my life because, like everyone else, I have bad days as well as good days.

Here's an example. A couple of years ago, I had a particularly tough day in A&E ahead of me. It was a Monday, I was tired and I wasn't feeling particularly motivated. I felt it was important to share that, so that among all the #starttheweekstrong and #motivationalmonday hashtags, there was a voice saying, 'Don't feel bad if you're not having a good day, it's okay and it happens to us all.' Just sharing that moment of 'meh' with my followers allowed others to do the same and I hope it made us all feel a little more connected to reality, rather than to some unachievable image of go-go-go. The core of social media is sharing; that means letting people in on the bad as well as the good.

WHAT'S THE WORST THAT CAN HAPPEN?

Failure is a process. The main thing to remember is that, like any stress response, failure generates thoughts that affect your feelings. If you struggle when something goes wrong, talk to someone, or try to do something that will help you unwind. Going for a run or a stomp (see page 40) can help with getting some perspective. Thanks to that early lesson my parents gave me, I now always ask myself, 'What's the worst that can happen?' And I guarantee, the reality is nowhere near as bad as you think it will be. It's such a simple tool, but so effective. Look at the worksheets Weaken Worry, Deal with Doom and Talk Thoughts (see pages 219, 220 and 227) for practical ways to help yourself, as well as Take Action – Friendly Failure (see page 94).

I used this 'What's the worst that can happen?' line recently when my friend Adam and I decided to go for our motorcycle driving tests. The nearer we got to the test date, the more nervous Adam became. He began coming up with reasons why he may as well just throw in the towel. The night before the test, he texted me to say he wasn't going. So I pulled out all the motivational energy I could find and asked him to consider the worst thing that could happen: that he would fail.

And if that happened, he could just sit the test again and would have learned from the mistakes he made first time around. After some time, Adam agreed that trying was worth it, even if he failed.

Next morning, we set off to the test centre. And do you know what happened? We both passed. In fact, a few weeks later the worst actually happened to me, not him. It was when I was taking the module 2 test: I made a silly mistake while turning and instantly knew I'd failed, but I also knew I'd never make that mistake again. One week later, I sat the test again and passed. And this time with an even bigger sense of achievement and some life lessons in my back pocket. Figure out the worst thing, then figure out how you will cope with it.

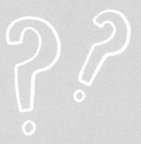

CHALLENGE THE NARRATIVE

WHAT'S BEHIND OUR WORRIES?

We live in a culture that worships perfection. Whether that's in school or university, at work or on social media, we are expected to be our best at all times. No wonder people develop a phobia about failing. And even when they do achieve, they can't enjoy it, because they're fearful of not being able to repeat their success. This has stopped many people from achieving the things they want.

As with many hang-ups, the roots of the fear of failure can be traced back to childhood. We all want to please our parents when we're kids – I know I did – but at some point, you have to let go of that need for validation. It can stand in the way of seeing tasks and goals objectively, making your efforts personalized and relating to your self-esteem rather than to your ability. If failing to do something is tied in to how you feel you're perceived by others, then it stands to reason you'll be less inclined to attempt projects in which you could potentially fall short.

We live curated lives. We tend only to hear about people's wins and successes. We don't see failure talked about very often and, when it is, it's usually framed as bad news. Again, there's a stigma attached to not achieving a goal that makes it something to be kept to yourself. When everyone else is shouting about their successes, this can be very isolating.

It's important to challenge this narrative. It's causing all of us to believe that others have their lives more together than we do. That we're alone in failing, or making mistakes. That others are achieving their goals on the first try, while we take multiple attempts to pull off what we're aiming for. Every time you think you have to reach for perfection, challenge that narrative. It's not reality. There's not a single person on the planet who hasn't made multiple mistakes while living a big and full life. It's just not possible. Stop expecting that of yourself, it's not realistic, nor healthy.

FRIENDLY FAILURE

I'm naturally an introverted person and there have definitely been times when the fear of failure has affected me, but I've learned to fail well. Part of that is finding positives in failure and taking confidence from it. A good example for me was when I missed out on my grades for med school. At first, I felt terrible, really awful, but in many ways that was a good thing because it showed I cared about my exams. It made me realize how much it meant to me. After that, I didn't take any chances. I used the experience to avoid putting myself in that position again. As hard as it seemed at the time, I had to accept that I'd messed up, go through the emotions, and formulate a plan.

I had to work out where I had gone wrong and what I could do to fix the situation. I planned how to get my place back – take a year out, study harder, retake my exams – and then moved forward. And it worked, too: I reapplied, did the course work, smashed the interview and soon found myself at med school facing a whole new set of challenges. But I had my experience of turning around a failure as evidence to combat any future self-doubt.

The next time fear of failure rears its ugly head in your direction, ask yourself the following questions and see if you can make a friend of it rather than a foe.

1. **What's the reason for your fear? Is there evidence to back it up?**

2. **What's the worst-case scenario? How likely is it to happen?**

3. **What's your contingency plan if things going wrong?**

4. **What's the best outcome?**

5. **Good or bad, what will you learn from the experience?**

STRIKE A POSE

If you're feeling a little wobbly before a presentation or test, I want to give you a tool that will bypass your brain and help with that fear of failure. It's to stand like a superhero. You might want to run to the bathroom to do this in private, but you'll be surprised at how quickly it'll boost your confidence and allow you to push on. How do you stand like a superhero? Stand with your legs hip-width apart, put your hands on your hips with your elbows sticking out and raise your chest up like you're Superman. If you look in the mirror, you'll see the pose has pulled your shoulders back, opened your lungs and given you a sense of strength that wasn't there before. Now, go forth and save the day!

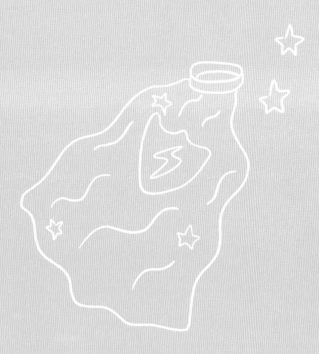

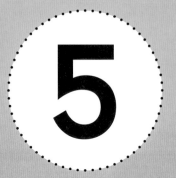

STRESS IS THE ENEMY

Chronic stress wreaks havoc on your body's physical and mental health. Release the idea that stress creates success and allow for a softer approach to life.

When was the last time you felt stressed out? Last week? Yesterday? Five minutes ago?

In this hectic day and age, feeling stressed is an accepted part of life. Some thrive on it, others try to avoid it, but we all experience it. Every day seems to bring new research showing us how people's anxiety levels are the highest they've ever been. The baseline has been raised and we are all living with ever-increasing levels of stress.

It's important that we create an environment within which we can handle stress when it appears. We need to meet it head on, to stop it creeping up on us when we're at a low ebb. In this chapter, I'll look at how to stay mentally agile, how to pre-empt our stressors through good emotional health and by being open about it, to stop stress having a corrosive effect on our sense of self. But before I start, it's important to remember that we *all* feel stressed at times. None of us is immune. And a little bit of stress can sometimes be good, as it can motivate us. But when things start to get on top of us, we tend to feel powerless and isolated. If there's one tip I can give when approaching stress, whatever the cause, it's to get it out in the open and talk to someone. A problem shared really is a problem halved, and by sharing your worries with another human being you'll find that you're not alone.

If you look at the statistical trends in mental illness, an increasing number of people who previously had mild depression and anxiety that they could basically manage themselves are now seeking a clinical diagnosis. That's compounded by those already in the system getting sicker, causing a massive increase in people seeking help and putting a strain on the health sector. And it seems to be hitting Gen Zs and Millennials hardest. My own doctor told me she's never seen so many people of this age on medication. And the biggest concerns for these two age groups are financial issues, job insecurity, concerns about mortality and what their future might look like. The year 2020 showed us that we truly have so little control over our lives; carrying that worry around with us on a daily basis is, understandably, causing problems.

CARRYING STRESS IN YOUR WALLET

The effects money concerns can have on mental health are both varied and cyclical. If people are struggling with their finances, it's likely to be detrimental to their wellbeing... and vice versa. But although we can't all make ourselves more financially secure – wouldn't that be nice? – there are things we can do to alleviate the anxieties that money worries can cause.

Before I talk about what we can do when we get into financial difficulty, there's something I want to get off of my chest. As the old saying goes, prevention is better than cure, so why aren't we taught about financial issues at school? If education is primarily about preparing children for adulthood, then shouldn't they be given the tools to navigate one of the most import areas of adult lives? There are many reasons why we work, but the main one is survival, to put a roof over our heads and food on the table. What we spend our money on is an everyday concern, so I really can't understand why financial basics – such as the differences between types of bank account, the essentials of savings and investments, the mechanics of rental agreements and mortgages – are not on the curriculum. Most kids don't have a clue and they take that ignorance with them into adulthood.

I was lucky. My mum worked in a bank, so she understood how important a basic understanding of financial terms was and shared her knowledge. But most people don't have a family member who works in finance, so they have to look to their parents (who themselves may not have much of an idea, as they weren't taught about money either), pay someone for financial advice, or wing it.

I'm convinced that one of the main reasons people get so stressed about money is because they don't understand it, feel stupid and embarrassed and bury their heads in the sand. In lieu of completely changing the education system, people need to know that, in the first instance, they can make an appointment at their local bank or Citizen's Advice office to speak to someone about financial issues. They won't tell you what to do with your money, but they will explain your options and help you understand what they mean. And once you have that knowledge, you can make a plan. Taking control of your money is one of the most empowering things you can do and will help alleviate the stress of financial uncertainty.

LOOKING AFTER THE PENNIES

Knowing about money is not the sole preserve of financial advisors and accountants, it's something that affects all of us every single day. And in that regard, a little bit of knowledge goes a very long way.

There are lots of great books out there that can help. One of my many self-help holiday reads was Emilie Bellet's *You're Not Broke, You're Pre-Rich* and I'd recommend it to anyone who wants to get a grip on their finances. What the book cleverly does is – very respectfully – treat the reader as a financial newbie and explain all the basics that I feel we should be taught at school. It's really accessible and certainly gave me a lot of things to think about regarding my own approach to money. It also identifies how feeling financially secure is key to mental health and wellbeing. While you might not think you have money to worry about right now, the fact that you don't is probably causing stress. Read up and calm any concerns you have.

Taking control of my finances got rid of anxiety that I didn't even realize I was carrying around. I come from a fairly modest background, where spare money was scarce; we couldn't afford to go on holiday or do a lot of things that my friends' families could do. When I started earnin money, finances were something I really worried about, especially the fact of having a student loan. I wanted to learn what my options were and how I could make what I earned work for me. Financial stress is horrible and I wanted to avoid it as much as possible.

TAKE BACK CONTROL

Having money worries is nothing to be ashamed of, but the thought of being judged stops a lot of us from asking for help. When people are faced with something they don't understand, they either get frightened or angry. It's not about blame, it's about talking to someone who can advise you. In the first instance, reaching out to family and friends can take a load off your mind. But if you need professional advice, charities such as StepChange or The Money Charity can offer free consultations, while your doctor is always there for anxiety issues, should they flare up.

One aspect of financial insecurity is the feeling of helplessness, of not having control over your own life. That powerlessness can be overwhelming, so look at what factors you *can* control. Whether it be making an honest account of your finances or contacting your creditors, just don't bury your head in the sand.

Be honest about your spending habits. If you buy things impulsively on your phone, remove all your bank details so they don't auto-fill: those extra seconds could be the difference between proceeding with an unnecessary purchase or not. Or if credit cards are your problem, try cutting them up and going cash only. Some people suggest putting credit cards in a bowl of water in the freezer, so you have to wait for a block of ice to defrost before using them, again putting a buffer between the impulse and the buy.

We tend not to talk about money in the UK; it makes people uncomfortable and worried that they'll come off badly by comparison. But as with so many of the issues I've shared with you, having an open and honest discussion about money would massively destigmatize the subject. It would help people identify where they have a problem and give them a forum to discuss what to do about it. If we don't take control of our money, it will take control of us. It's as simple as that.

SPHERE OF INFLUENCE

When we were 14, my best friend Adam shared with me an incredible tool that his dad taught him. It's called the Sphere of Influence and it's all about control. There are things we have control over, such as how we spend our money, what we eat and who we speak to. Then there are things we have no control over, such as how others react, what other people think of us, or whether our favourite sports team will win. The thing is, we worry about both categories. We spread our energy across them in the hopes of figuring out a way that we can get in control. And while this makes sense for the first category, it doesn't for the second.

For the Sphere of Influence tool, I want you to draw a huge circle on a page (see page 226 for a template). Then, inside the circle, write out all the things you can control. Fill it up with any many of your worries as possible, but only the ones that you have the power to do something about. Now, outside the circle, write all the things you cannot control, where the outcome is in someone else's hands. Anything that's outside the circle – or the Sphere of Influence – is outside of your control, so drop any worry you have about it. If you try this exercise, you'll realize it switches something in your brain, where you realize that the worry is pointless. You can put down those concerns and dedicate your energy to the things you can take care of.

Formula One drivers exemplify this perfectly. Before a race, each of the 20 drivers (and their teams) will have readied themselves and their car for the twists and turns of the tarmac. They will have put together a plan for what they can control, such as when to take a pitstop or which tyres to use, and – more importantly – they will have prepared for what they cannot control. The driver ahead of them may crash and suddenly they'll have to swerve to avoid a collision. Perhaps the weather starts to heat up and the track becomes too hot for the soft tyres, well then, they'll go into the pits to change tyres. There are many factors the drivers can't control, but they can prepare themselves to cope when challenges occur. This is how I like to look at the Sphere of Influence. If I can't control it, I don't worry about it, because I trust myself enough to overcome whatever happens.

It doesn't matter how slowly you move, as long as you don't stop.

THE STRESS WE SEEK – DOOMSCROLLING

When I was younger, we only had one TV in the house, so we'd all watch the soaps – *EastEnders* and *Coronation Street* – religiously as a family. But when I got to about 17 or 18, I realized that it was all so miserable, so I just stopped watching soaps entirely and never went back.

I think about that a lot in relation to doomscrolling, that addictive engagement with endlessly grim content on our devices. Like the drama of soap opera plotlines, bad news triggers us psychologically, so we keep coming back for more. The excitement we feel when new information arrives is in fact a release of the hormone dopamine (known as the 'reward' chemical), which we're programmed to respond to. However, that doesn't mean it's good for us.

As a species, we're hardwired to react to perceived threats and the apps we use account for this. The algorithms that control our news feeds take this tendency to focus on bad news and supercharge it. Reading or watching bad news alerts our fight-or-flight response – which is there primarily to protect us from danger – in the same way that grim TV soaps do. The difference is that an episode of *EastEnders* comes to an end, but 24-hour social media and news feeds don't. On our devices, the misery is endless. If our brains don't get a chance to rest from reacting to all this stimulation, we start to suffer stress-related symptoms.

DIGITAL CLEANSE

There can be so much bad news around that it puts us all in danger of burnout. If we feel our mood is being affected, then it's time to take a serious look at our digital media consumption. I'm not talking about deleting all our apps and cutting ourselves off from the world; feeling isolated is just as bad for our mental health as being over-stimulated. But we need to know where the tipping point is: the line between knowing enough about what's going on in the world and knowing so much that it causes anxiety.

A few years ago, I deleted my Twitter account. I wasn't being trolled, I just found that most of what I saw on the platform was negative and demotivating. Now that I've deleted it, I find that I don't even miss it, but I certainly value the reduction of stress and negativity in my day. Is there some app you can do this with? Is there something that adds more negativity than positivity to your life? If so, consider what you value more: the app or your mental health.

CREATE YOUR OWN SCHEDULE

When I was a kid, newspapers could only carry so much information and the news on TV was only broadcast a couple of times a day. If you're showing signs of overload, then I suggest designing a schedule for your daily news consumption. Also, seek out and engage with positive news stories on your favourite social media platforms, which will reshape your personal algorithm. If you're seen to be looking at good news, the platforms will send you notifications for more. There are plenty of positive news websites and feeds you can follow, but think about alternatives such as signing up to positive newsletters, subscribing to non-news podcasts, or watching comedy, as a way to remind yourself it's not all bad.

And think about content beyond your devices too. As someone who has seen the aftermath of tragic events first-hand in a hospital emergency department, I find the popularity of real-life murder and accident documentaries baffling. There are plenty of life-affirming shows out there, things that will lift your mood rather than challenge your nervous system. Even if you can't resist the latest true crime series, find a feelgood show to balance it out. Carve out time for what makes you feel good and stops you overthinking.

TAKE TIME TO GRIEVE

Grief is a difficult and challenging process and everyone deals with it differently. For me, when I lost my little brother, I tried to rush back to normality as quickly as possible. I was literally back at work four days after it happened. That was initially my way of dealing with it. But I came to realize that the reason there are stages of grief is that they need to be worked through. Now I know I'm still working through them. What's particularly hard with Llŷr is that I never had a chance to say goodbye. One minute he was alive, then I took a call and found out he wasn't.

While we may have an inkling when some people are going to pass – the elderly or those who have a terminal condition – we never really know when exactly that moment will come. In that way, every death comes as a shock. But if you do have an opportunity to prepare for it, take it. Make time to write down everything you want to say to that person and find the time to meet up with them and *say it*, so when it happens, you'll have told them what you wanted to.

And when the time comes, make sure you give yourself space to process the loss and grieve in your own time. We need to move away from this idea of needing to 'get over a bereavement'. You never get over it, you just learn to live with it. In 40 years' time, I'm not going to think it's any less sad that Llŷr died, or miss him any less. I may have learned to live with it with greater ease, but I'm never going to 'get over it'. And that's okay.

Whether you need to be with other people while you grieve, or you prefer to be alone, you must do whatever works best for you. But make sure you invest in the process of healing. I would recommend therapy if you're struggling, but be aware that the timing needs to be right. It took more than a year after Llŷr's passing until I felt I was ready for therapy, before that it wouldn't have worked for me. Take your time, because as individuals we approach everything in different ways and grief is no different. It's your journey, do it your way.

Only those who truly care about you will hear you when you are quiet.

WE ONLY GET ONE LIFE

Death is a difficult topic to talk about and any loss never truly leaves us. But, as with all the issues I've talked about in this chapter, there are positives to be found, although inevitably tinged with sadness in this case. A life lived well is a life worth celebrating, and the memories of a lost loved one can lift and inspire us in many ways. We would be doing the dead a disservice if the pain of their passing stopped us from remembering the good times shared and enjoying the life we still have.

Even before Llŷr passed, I was looking at how I could be of use in the youth mental health space. In fact, he and I talked about it a lot. Everything I've done as the UK government's Youth Mental Health Ambassador and with the youth mental health charity HEADucation has been inspired by my little brother, and of course he was an important part of my BBC Children in Need documentary too.

And while our own mortality isn't something we may want to dwell upon too much, an awareness of it can help us get more out of our lives. It can help us cherish those closest to us, keep us mindful of wasting time, let us be thankful for what we have and allow us to live in the present. I feel grateful for every day I have and feel inspired by the memory of my brother to make the most of it, whether that be helping others, spending time with friends and family, or just being happy. We only have one shot at this, so let's all make the most of it.

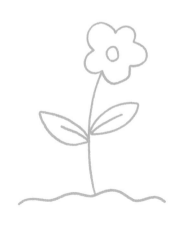

REWRITE YOUR CAREER PATH

When many of us think of work, we think of stress. For Gen Zs and Millennials, the worries appear to be multi-layered. From concerns over unemployment and job security, to our inconsistent career paths and their effect on our financial wellbeing, whole generations are living with a pervasive undercurrent of stress.

It's important to remember that our jobs aren't only a way of making the money we need to live, they're a reflection of who and where we are in life. Losing a job you love, or having one you don't like, can have a massive effect on your self-esteem and sense of self. But there is light at the end of the tunnel, you've just got to reassess and reframe your work.

Since the dawn of the industrial age, technological advances have made life easier for us, year after year. And while our parents may have experienced a slower change in the pace of life, we unfortunately don't have that luxury. For many of us, the jobs we expected to pursue when we left school may not exist anymore. You might have gone into a career expecting to do X, Y and Z, but all the changes of recent years have meant that role or industry has completely changed into one that you no longer have an interest in pursuing.

Change can be difficult, but we need to be fearless in the face of it. I'm not talking about bravery or courage, but rather being fear-less, not trapped by fear.

Your parents probably grew up with the idea of a 'job for life'. These days, we all have to be more flexible. You may have several strands to your career, or several careers over the years. Versatility, skill transference and being open to change are commendable traits to have when it comes to the job market.

And if you have to make a pivot – or even a U-turn – along the way, then it's not like you're starting from scratch, as you take all the experience you've gained previously with you. All those skills and all that knowledge can be applied to your next adventure, in life as well as in your work.

When change is inevitable, ask yourself that much-loved question of mine: 'What's the worst that can happen?' It bears repeating. If you take a couple of minutes to think carefully about what could be the absolute worst-case scenario of any given situation, you'll soon find that it's either not as bad as you think or that it's highly unlikely to end up that way. Visualizing the possibilities in advance can help to diffuse some of your anxiety around them.

DEALING WITH DEATH

Nobody wants to think about death. It can trigger stress even when it remains a hypothetical state. Whether it's a member of our family, or someone we know, a pet, or even ourselves, we don't want to consider the fact that we are going lose people and they are no longer going to be in our lives. But the harsh reality is that death is inevitable: we are all going to die. Working in A&E, I saw death on a regular basis. Heart attacks or traffic accidents are shocking and sudden and leave people with unanswered questions. And during the pandemic, it was hard to see the sheer number of people who passed away, as well as their families having to process it.

Losing someone close to us can be devastating, and grief – the collection of emotions we go through following a bereavement – can be difficult and painful to navigate. There's no right or wrong way to grieve. It's different for everyone, and the symptoms of grief are varied. It's said that there are seven stages of grief: shock or disbelief, denial, bargaining, guilt, anger, depression, then acceptance combined with – in most cases – hope. These are experienced almost universally and almost always in that order, according to psychiatrist Elisabeth Kübler-Ross in her book *On Death and Dying*.

As a medic, I can say that in the UK we hide away from death and we're pretty awful at dealing with grief. I'm not suggesting we dwell on it all the time, that would be equally unhealthy. Anxiety about death is a recognized condition – thanatophobia – and is a common symptom of other mental illnesses. It can be extremely debilitating. But an awareness of death may stop us walking around thinking we're invincible, which we're not, and also prepare us in a small way for the inevitable.

Something else we're pretty bad at is supporting other people through grief. Obviously, this isn't intentional, it's just another aspect of death not being part of the general conversation. In my experience good practice isn't *offering* to help, it's just going out and *doing* it. People who are grieving don't know what they need, especially for the first few weeks when they're in shock. They may not be sleeping, they may forget to eat. If you know someone who's in that position, don't wait to ask, just do.

HARNESS YOUR STRESS

Remember that from an evolutionary perspective, stress is there to protect us, to prevent us from getting into situations that cause us harm. It isn't necessarily a negative: being stressed just means we're alive. It's how we react to it that dictates whether stress helps or hinders us. How we frame stress is the most important factor.

Stress is the body's way of sending us a very simple message: take action. If your finances are causing you worry, seek advice. If you're unhappy at work, look for new opportunities. If social media is causing you anxiety, delete the apps. These actions may not completely change how you're feeling, or solve your problems, but they're a start. In many ways, stress is an early warning signal, letting us know things are getting too much. Take action – no matter how small – because it can make a big difference.

NO TIME LIKE NOW

DARE TO SHARE

Share a worry with someone right now. Send a text, make a phone call, post it on your socials if you feel the call. A problem shared is a problem halved. Watch how quickly it turns from a mountain into a molehill when you share it.

YOU ARE ENOUGH

When you define what really matters to you, rather than what matters to others, you'll realize that you have value and that you always did. Your life is worth its weight in gold.

Do you sometimes feel that any success you achieve is down to good luck? Do you feel guilt instead of pride when you accomplish something great? Are you unable to accept compliments because you feel you're close to being exposed as a fraud? If so, then you're one of many people who experience the self-limiting effects of impostor syndrome.

In my experience, impostor syndrome manifests as self-undermining internal statements, such as 'Should I really be doing this?' 'Do I deserve this?' 'Am I going to get found out?' It's a form of self-doubt that stems from a feeling of not being *enough*. Good enough, attractive enough, smart enough ... pick a category, you'll just feel not-enough in it. And when it comes to your mental fitness, that can be really damaging.

The ironic thing is this: people who suffer *most* from impostor syndrome work really hard and go above and beyond to get the job done. Yet they still tend to devalue their efforts. They make up for their self-perceived 'lack of talent' with charm, self-depreciation or other subservient behaviours, including working unnecessarily long hours or undervaluing their financial worth. Despite this excessive perfectionism, they still experience that self-doubt and low self-worth. It's a cycle that's very hard to break free from. Psychologist Audrey Ervin, who has written extensively about the condition, describes potential sufferers as 'anyone who isn't able to internalize and own their success'. I believe that's all of us, to some extent, at some point.

Impostor syndrome was identified more than 40 years ago by psychologists Dr Pauline Rose Clance and Dr Suzanne Imes. At first it was thought only to affect women working in predominantly male environments, but over time, it was discovered that similar feelings were being experienced by the BAME community, lower-income groups and people with disabilities. These days it's widely accepted that impostor syndrome can be experienced by just about anyone. Those feelings of being revealed as a fraud, or feeling shame about your achievements, are universal. It's estimated that 70 per cent of us will experience them during our lives.[15] And if you're one of them, let me help.

WHAT TYPE ARE YOU?

In her book *The Secret Thoughts of Successful Women*, Dr Valerie Young identifies the types of people who are susceptible to impostor syndrome:

Perfectionists – even if they meet 99 per cent of their goals, they still feel like failures.

Experts – feel the need to know everything and constantly seek affirmation through new qualifications and training.

Natural geniuses – when effort is required, they feel like they're failing.

Soloists – don't ask for help and feel like a fraud if they need to ask.

Superwomen/men – overachievers who have to constantly strive to avoid feeling fake.

The behaviours displayed by these different types vary but can also overlap (for example, I identify with a couple of these classifications and display traits from both of them). A perfectionist will respond badly to the slightest mistake and use that as justification for their impostor feelings, while superwomen/men will overcompensate by working harder than anyone else to prove they're not fraudulent. If you identify with any of these behaviours at all, the thing they have in common is that they can affect the quality of your life, not just at work but outside of it too. It can result in burnout, anxiety and depression.

I don't want to make it sound like I've got my impostor syndrome completely sorted. I may have ways of dealing with the feelings, but when they strike it can still make things very difficult. Earlier, I spoke about my anxiety and, unfortunately for me, the physical manifestation of impostor syndrome presents itself in this way. My thoughts will race and I'll start to question my ability to achieve the things I want.

When this happens, the first step I take is to try and calm my mind and reassure myself. One technique that works for me is to identify a previous time I felt this way and look at the event that made me anxious back then. Maybe it was my first day on the ward as a junior doctor, or my *Love Island* audition, whatever, it's usually an incident where I felt impossibly out of my depth. Once I've visualized that, I'll think, 'Well, you managed to get through that challenge and nothing bad happened, so there's no reason why you can't deal with what's in front of you, Alex.'

Impostor syndrome centres around the idea that you're not up to the job. So, I look for evidence from my past that shows that yes, I am up to the task, whether that be speaking in front of huge groups of people, presenting my own documentary, or simply facing up to a tough week (see the Gather Evidence worksheet on page 224).

My role as a Youth Mental Health Ambassador for the UK government is probably my biggest trigger of impostor syndrome. And it's sometimes been cruelly reinforced by people who've not been shy about telling me that they think I'm a fraud, too. As you can imagine, that makes the feelings even harder to process: other people agreeing with your inner critic! That's when I really need to take a step back and remind myself why I took on the role in the first place. I have to look for that evidence and reinstate my belief that, even if it's just in a small way, I'm adding value to people's lives with what I'm doing.

That's my best piece of advice if this happens to you. It doesn't matter what your circumstance or what you're doing, when that inner critic strikes, bring yourself back to the present moment and focus on the task in hand. A lot of the time, impostor syndrome is simply worrying about what could happen in the future rather than focusing on what's happening now. You are never going to be 100 per cent ready and it's never going to be exactly the right time. But that's the point. It means every moment is the right moment. If you want it, you just have to do it.

Another thing to consider is that nearly everyone suffers from impostor syndrome at some point in their lives. When I was a med student, I was looking at final year students and thinking how confident they looked... and yet, when I reached that point, I still felt like an impostor. I've had veteran consultants tell me that, after 18 years in practice, they still go home, sit in their pyjamas watching Netflix and question whether they're really up to the task of being a doctor. It's good to know, but also highlights how prevalent these feelings of inadequacy really are.

HOW TO TURN IMPOSTOR SYNDROME
INTO EXPERT CONFIDENCE

When I feel like an impostor, I…

Acknowledge the thought.

Assess whether it's
toxic or constructive.

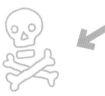 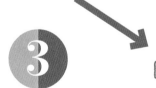 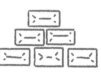

If it's toxic, I find
evidence and then
I negate it.

If it's constructive,
I discover my knowledge
gaps and then I act.

THE IMPOSTOR WITHIN

Personally, I've always felt like a bit of an impostor, and several events in my life seemed to validate that for me. I didn't have an easy time at school; I was quite bright, but I had undiagnosed dyslexia (I was only formally diagnosed at medical school). I used to really struggle with traditional learning and had a very short attention span. This fed into my feelings of inadequacy and, despite knowing even as a child that I wanted a career in medicine, my grades and general standing academically made me wonder if I was capable.

I did manage to turn everything around by the time I left school, but again my impostor syndrome went into overdrive when I was applying for med school. I'd done my work experience at Morriston Hospital in Swansea and also got my place at Liverpool Medical School lined up. But when I received my A-level results, I'd missed out on my chemistry pass by two marks and had to redo the course work and reapply.

Looking back, I believe that negative became a positive. The fear of failing again drove me on, and five years later I left med school with a distinction, in the top 1 per cent in the country. Reframing failure can turn impostor syndrome from something debilitating into a motivation.

But before I reached that realization, I had to struggle with my inner critic throughout med school. Many of my fellow students had one or both parents who were doctors and that just added to my feeling of not belonging.

Even when I'd graduated and started working as a doctor, I'd sometimes catch myself thinking, 'I'm just this Welsh boy from Carmarthen and I'm here at King's College Hospital, with all these bright people!' I constantly felt as if I was going to get 'found out'.

You might have expected those feelings to follow me to *Love Island* but, oddly enough, they didn't. It was only after leaving the show that impostor syndrome set in once more. The level of attention I got, the increase in social media followers, people wanting to talk to me and take pictures, I just couldn't understand why they were interested. I found it very, very odd. In a funny way, any impostor syndrome I experienced at this time was justified – after all I wasn't an entertainer or a celebrity or a model. And I've no doubt that's why I always knew I'd return to medicine, where my true purpose lay.

THE INNER CRITIC

Whether self-identifying or looking out for a friend, here are some of the thought processes experienced by people in the throes of impostor syndrome. Do you recognize any of these traits in yourself or others? If so, it could be time to reach out for help.

- **Expert** – 'I need to know absolutely everything about this project before I can even think about working on it.'

- **Perfectionist** – 'Even the tiniest mistake proves I'm unsuitable to do this.'

- **Natural Genius** – 'Why, if I'm so talented, am I struggling?'

- **Soloist** – 'If I ask for help, that just proves I'm not up to the task.'

- **Superwoman/man** – 'I have to work harder than anyone else to make sure they don't find out I'm a fraud.'

MANAGING IMPOSTOR SYNDROME AT WORK

The workplace is the ideal breeding ground for self-doubt and feelings of being a fraud. But if you take a step back and look at how you approach your workload, criticism and relationships in the workplace can go some way to understanding your trigger points and how to manage them. Copy this list into your phone, or on to a sticky note on your screen, and refer to it when anxiety bites.

Set realistic goals.

Recognize your expertise.

Keep away from toxic competition.

Define what success means to you, not what it means to others.

Don't rely on external validation.

Set work limits and boundaries to avoid overwork.

Practice your response to failure.

Praise yourself for effort and success.

Ask for help.

Remember: nobody is perfect.

Nobody has it all figured out. That's the point! Life is exciting because the future is never certain.

OWN YOUR BEHAVIOURS

I'm a perfectionist. I like to get everything right. Even something as tiny as the title of the thumbnail on a YouTube video must be perfect. Yet I also find myself questioning whether I'm working hard enough and achieving as much as I can: typical superwoman/man behaviour. I have to try and control those urges and thoughts, and part of that is understanding *why* I feel that way.

As with most behaviours, it has roots in your societal and personal surroundings. Sometimes a belief system that you've inherited from your family or those who care for you means that you feel you're falling short of the mark.

I remember my mum being an absolute perfectionist when I was younger. She was very keen for my brothers and me to do well academically. I think this was because she didn't go to university and she wanted that for us. And although she didn't push us into any particular area – her whole approach was to urge us to do well at something we liked – she insisted we work hard at it and make sure we were the best. No pressure then! The three of us reacted to this in very different ways, but while it served us all well in the long run, I can see how I evolved into a perfectionist who always thinks they need to do more. Thanks Mum!

Joking aside, it does have its benefits. A good example of this was doing a personal training course when I was working in emergency medicine. I felt at the time that there was a gap in my knowledge when it came to talking about physical fitness and I was worried that someone might call me out on it. It was playing on my mind, so I thought the best way to deal with it was to get a qualification. I can see now that the root of it was impostor syndrome, but I took that niggling feeling and turned it into a positive by getting qualified as a personal trainer.

That's what I mean about reframing your feelings and using them as a positive force, rather than a negative one. I believe that having a little bit of self-doubt and admitting there are gaps in your knowledge is absolutely fine and, in some ways, essential for self-development. But rather than worrying about what people are going to think of you, go away and actually *do* something to mitigate your perceived gap. It may not completely negate the feeling of being a fraud, but at least you can take a step back and use it as evidence to prove you are capable when those feelings strike.

PREPARATION OFFERS RELIEF

I'm aware that this sounds like I'm having a constant inner conversation with myself. I'm not, but I *am* someone who's aware of upcoming triggers. That way I can prepare for any issues or 'what ifs' and make sure they don't catch me off guard. For example, not long ago I spoke at the Cheltenham Literary Festival and I knew it was going to cause me a bit of anxiety. Negative thoughts about whether I would be able to remain calm, or whether anyone would turn up to the Q&A. Or, if they did, would they be disparaging about my book, because I'm not a proper author... blah blah blah... really mentally exhausting stuff!

I let those thoughts go through my mind for a few moments and then said to myself, 'People responded really well to your book. You're talking about something that matters to you and that you think other people will be interested in, because it's an important topic'. And when I went out for the Q&A, the tent was full and the audience responded well and asked some genuinely interesting questions. After the talk, when I walked around the corner to the book signing area, there was a queue all the way out of the door!

While I'm aware that external validation shouldn't be your only way of finding value, in that instance it went a long way to quieting my inner voice. It also gave me evidence to store up to help shut the voice down when it returns in the future. Because it will – I know that – so I need to be ready for it. I'm a firm believer that the best way to deal with 'what ifs' is action, and for me that action is making sure I'm prepared.

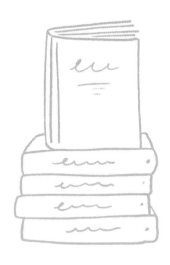

IMPOSTOR OR IMPROVER?

As I hope I've demonstrated, the negative feelings caused by impostor syndrome can be reframed and used to spur us on to greater achievements. My take on this isn't an exact science, but happily there is actual research out there that bears it out.

Recent studies carried out at the Massachusetts Institute of Technology found that impostor syndrome could actually motivate those experiencing it to perform better.[16] The study groups – one of which, coincidentally, consisted of late-stage medical students – found there was no significant difference in competence between those who felt like a fraud and those who did not. In fact, the impostors put extra effort into their communication skills. They outperformed their more confident colleagues in interpersonal skills. Despite the uncomfortable nature of impostor syndrome, it can be seen as a motivation rather than a sign of failure.

That's why I want to rebrand impostor syndrome as a superpower. Hopefully, the tips I've given here will help you see it can be a friend not a foe. But before we can make that shift, I think we need to be kinder to ourselves in general. People are so critical of themselves these days, myself included, and I think we need to make our inner voice a kinder one. Celebrate our successes, all of them, not just the big ones. Little victories, even things like getting the washing done or paying a bill,

are achievements that shouldn't go unnoticed. Sometimes it's hard enough to get through the day as it is, so giving yourself a pat on the back can make a small, incremental difference to your overall confidence.

And with confidence comes the ability to control that inner voice. Is what it's saying to you helpful? If so, great – use that to improve, to achieve, to be happier with yourself. But if it's not, shut it down, ignore it if you can. Use the evidence you've collected from your past achievements to prove it wrong. Your inner voice should be helping you, not hindering you. It's about time we turned impostor syndrome on its head and start seeing it as improver syndrome.

HAVE AN IMPOSTOR *MOMENT*, NOT AN IMPOSTOR LIFE

If you can reframe impostor syndrome and turn it on its head, then it can be a powerful tool for personal progress. Sure, qualifications-wise, I may not have seemed the most likely candidate for the role I have. I'm not a psychologist, nor do I have professional experience of working specifically with young people. But what I do have, through my own personal experience, is an understanding of young people's mental health issues and a desire to see change in the way they're treated, as well as strong views.

Even after all the work I've done so far, I still get that voice creeping in sometimes, saying, for instance, 'You haven't got a PhD in psychology and you're not a professor.' But rather than let that hinder me, I use it to spur me on. If I don't have those things, I ask myself what I *do* have. And when I take a step back and look at what I'm doing, I can see that, yes, I am achieving something and I am doing good. Sometimes engaging with your impostor syndrome can be a great motivator. It's even spurred me on to sign up to study a master's degree in Public Mental Health. And I love that it has. I've decided to follow the advice from Dr Valerie Young, expert in the field: 'Have an impostor moment, not an impostor life.'

WHAT TO DO WHEN IMPOSTOR SYNDROME STRIKES

Acknowledge

Allow the negative thoughts to sit with you, but only for a moment. You need to be aware that the thoughts exist, but not give them the time to have an effect.

Reframe

Think about what these thoughts are saying. Are they constructive, perhaps pointing out a genuine gap in your knowledge? Or are they destructive, toxic, self-limiting? If it's the former, then identifying areas requiring clarification or learning shows wisdom and self-knowledge. If it's the latter, move on to the next step.

Gather evidence

Remembering times when you have successfully negotiated an event that caused you anxiety will help you to negate self-doubt. Reminding yourself of qualifications or experience that prove you're up to the task can help to assuage negative thoughts. Keeping a list in the notes of your phone gives you something tangible to turn to in times of need.

Externalize

As the saying goes, a problem shared is a problem halved, and that goes for impostor syndrome too. While seeking external validation isn't ideal, when it comes to moments of anxiety, seeking reassurance from a friend or colleague can give you an outside perspective that breaks the internal echo chamber of self-doubt.

Celebrate your successes

There's nothing wrong with taking the time to look back at your wins and savour them. Instead of being your own worst critic, be your own cheerleader instead. Forget all this nonsense about being humble and self-effacing; if you've achieved something that you're proud of, shout about it! Even if you don't feel comfortable doing that publicly, do it for yourself. Print out the email your boss sent you telling you how well you're doing. Hang your school/college/training certificate on the wall. Then store these successes away mentally for the next time that inner voice tries to undermine you.

NAME YOUR IMPOSTOR

It may sound a little silly, but I suggest giving your impostor syndrome a name. This is great for times when it pops up, so you can differentiate it from yourself and your healthy thoughts. The sillier the name, the better, because it'll lessen its power over you. Eventually, you'll be ready to say, 'Oh, here's Mr Tiddlywinks again, trying to tell me I'm no good...' That doesn't sound too threatening now, does it?

~~Negative Nelly~~

~~Fretsome Frank~~

~~Silly Susan~~

~~Worrying William~~

MR TIDDLYWINKS

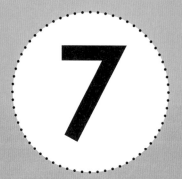

HAPPINESS IS
AN INSIDE JOB

If you are chasing happiness through a job,
a relationship or a new pair of trainers, you're
in for disappointment. True peace can't be
outsourced.

You would be forgiven for thinking that happiness is something that's found outside yourself. It's easy to assume when you wake up not happy and in a bad mood, or a bout of depression has set in, that – surely – you need to source happiness externally. Thankfully, though, this is not true. Happiness is something you harness within yourself, not something you tack on to you like some kind of medal.

The dictionary defines happiness as 'a state of wellbeing and contentment', which sounds very reasonable and yet not particularly exciting. Surely happiness means uncontrollable joy, jumping around with a huge smile on your face? Isn't that what society would have us believe, that happiness is a constant state brought on by owning a dream home, buying a new car, indulging in an expensive holiday? Basically, you'd be forgiven for assuming that the acquisition of 'stuff' is the path to true happiness. It's not.

Our brains (and society) will try to convince us that happiness is the state we should be in all of the time and that, if we're not, we're somehow failing at this thing called life. But, as we now know, we should be aiming for peace, not happiness, as a baseline (see page 8). Peace is the happy median. Choosing peace allows us space to add a little 'happy' in, as if it was the sprinkles on a cake. And when we do that, we release the need to chase the constant high. Let's look at some ways to add those sprinkles to your life.

THE MONEY TRAP

You've heard the saying: money can't buy happiness. And while that is true, more money can certainly make life easier. Having a roof over your head and food on the table is going to reduce the worry and stress that can lead to anxiety and depression. It expands the choices we can make for our lives and frees us up from basic survival concerns. Without a doubt, financial stability helps mental stability.

Our capitalist culture uses psychology and marketing to tap into that need for security, by convincing us that we can never have enough. That, if we just had more money, life would be better. It whizzes past our survival needs and tries to convince us that status counts just as much. Our status becomes connected to our survival, and, as we are creatures of community and belonging, we consider any potential threat to our status as a risk. As if we could be banished out into the wild, like our hunter-gatherer ancestors before us. Of course, we won't, but that doesn't stop the endless streams of adverts telling us that we need more. We are told that more money will get us more things, and more things will secure our status, and then we'll be happy. Safe. Only it's never-ending. You can never have enough under this model. It's manufactured that way intentionally – it's not called consumerism for nothing. But the interesting thing is that we have proof it doesn't work. Scientific proof.

You may be surprised to find that financial happiness has a limit. A US study carried out in 2010, which aimed to correlate wellbeing with salary, found that $75k (about £50k at the time, but over £60k with current exchange rates) is the sweet spot when it comes to earnings.[17] At every increment up until you hit that amount, your life measurably improves. But earn any more than that and, while life may get easier in some ways, the effect is considerably less profound. The reasons for this are unclear, although it has been suggested that too much wealth undercuts happiness levels because the more money you have, the less you appreciate what it brings you.

BIG BUCKS, BIG STRESS

A friend of mine, let's call him Toby, is in his late 20s and has always worked ridiculously hard, toiling away long hours, weekdays, weekends and evenings. Sure, he earns a lot of money and has all the benefits of that, but what he doesn't have is the time to enjoy any of it or spend quality time with his friends and family. I've spoken to him countless times and asked him to slow down, but he never has. Although recently he has started to question his habits, so my persistence may be paying off!

It's hard to convince someone who gets their self-worth from always being on the go and earning money that slowing down and taking time for themselves is the true path to happiness. This comes down to identifying your true motivations and shifting your focus to them. Think of it as having an inner and outer 'scorecard'. Are you more interested in having a high score that no one can see, or a low score that everyone can? Comparing yourself to others won't make you happy, but making sure you're fulfilled on the inside will.

The most powerful drug in the world is kindness.

THE SCIENCE OF HAPPINESS

Considering the quest for happiness has been around since the dawn of time, it's not surprising that there's a whole wing of science devoted to discovering the secret to what makes happy people happy.

The scientific study of happiness, sometimes called positive psychology, can be traced back to the late 1980s and the work of Mihaly Csikszentmihalyi (pronounced 'me-hi cheek-send-me-high'). He was a Hungarian-American psychologist who pioneered the concept of 'flow', a highly focused mental state conducive to productivity. Csikszentmihalyi believed that happiness is an intrinsic state of being and not an extrinsic one (which means it comes from within, it doesn't come from the external world). He believed that people have some degree of control over their happiness, although it takes a committed effort.

There have been many studies carried out over the years in which happiness has been measured under scientific conditions, using methods such as questionnaires, stress hormone (cortisol) measurements, and even social media analysis. I recently heard about the work of Professor Laurie Santos, known as the 'Happiness Professor', who runs The Science of Wellbeing course at Yale University in the US. It's one of the most popular courses in the university's history and her research points to the importance of feeling socially connected for improving happiness.

Professor Santos points out the tendency to think of happiness as a destination. We think once we've 'arrived there' we remain in that state, but she says that's the wrong approach. Rather, she points to happiness as a combination of factors that we need to work at continuously to maintain. She has a great metaphor about happiness being like a 'leaky tyre' that's slowly going down and needs to be continually inflated. And according to Santos, one of the key elements for keeping our happiness pumped up is social interaction.

THE HAPPIEST PEOPLE ON EARTH

It seems that the strongest link to happiness comes from a sense of belonging and generosity to others. Those who practice the following behaviours have been shown to be the happiest:

Express gratitude.

Show kindness.

Belong to a community.

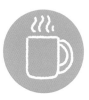

Volunteer their time.

Stay mindful.

Move their bodies.[18]

I AM GRATEFUL FOR...

Rolo for saving my mental health when he first arrived, through unconditional love and joy.

Trees and grass and birds and nature as a whole, which makes me feel even more alive when I am out walking in it.

My parents and my brother who have gone over and above to support me in every way possible. To tell me when I'm right, tell me when I'm wrong. They are amazing.

My body. I'm so grateful that, other than a few aches and pains, my body allows me to do everything I want to do in this life.

The time I have on this earth. I will never take any of it for granted.

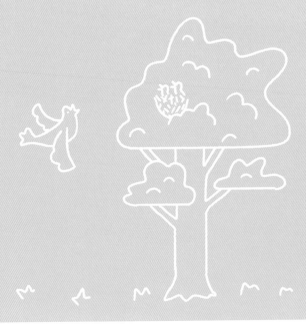

Just because someone
is doing it differently
to you, doesn't mean you
are doing it wrong.

COMPARISON IS THE THIEF OF JOY

Countless research papers have proven this old adage true, but never has it been more apparent than now. Comparison is the joy thief of the 21st century. We spend more of our lives comparing ourselves to others than any generation before us. These days, we are not just 'keeping up with the Joneses' next door, but with the Joneses in the next city, country, continent.

Social comparison is known to be negatively linked to increased depression and anxiety. And is it any wonder? Social media has curated out the hard times that each of us face, creating a false impression that all is well with everyone but us. What happens is that we compare the behind-the-scenes version of ourselves with the Insta-ready version of everyone else, meaning we always come up short.

When it comes to protecting your joy, there are two things to remember. Firstly, the curated socials are not real life, you are not the only person living through challenging times. Everyone does at some point in their lives. And secondly, you have the power to shut it out. The only person you should compare yourself to is you. If you think your childhood self would be proud of the person you've become, then clap yourself on the back. If you think that child-you might wish you'd done more, then consider doing it. Keep that kid in mind and ignore the rest; nobody's journey is more important to you than the one you're on.

THE BEST THINGS IN LIFE AREN'T THINGS

Something on which the happiness experts all agree is that our intuition as to what makes us happy is often wrong. It would be nice if our brain pointed us towards true contentment, but it has to compete with the ease of an online purchase or the dopamine hit of 'likes' on social media. When we use anything outside of ourselves to quench our thirst for happiness, we end up with the opposite. It's important to challenge the narrative that happiness is something we buy. It's not, so stop wasting your money.

I have come to believe, though, that we can train our minds to seek out the *right* forms of happiness. It's just a matter of figuring out what those are for you. It comes down to our personal values, those principles that matter more to us than anything else. When we align our lives to our values, everything improves. Perhaps you're someone who believes family is more important than anything else. So, if you move halfway across the world, away from family, you are unlikely to feel happy until you either build a family of your own or relocate back home. Conversely, if you value adventure and novelty, then a job-for-life that offers nothing but routine is not for you. It's important to know these values, to understand that sometimes what other people want – for you or for themselves – is not actually what you want for you.

A while back I got chatting to the nurse doing my lateral flow test on set. She told me that she'd been a London bus driver for 35 years. For the first ten of those, it was the best job she'd ever had. She'd got to know the regulars on her route; it was very sociable and she felt part of the community. But when screens and cashless payment cards were introduced to protect the drivers in their cabs, she suddenly found that she couldn't connect with her passengers. Even though hundreds of people passed her every day, she started to feel lonely and isolated and, in the end, had to leave the job. Her values were no longer being met. The interaction with her passengers meant more to her than any other part of the job. And now, as a nurse, chatting away to the likes of me, she's back in her element: connecting with her community.

When it comes to values, we will likely have a long list of things that are important to us. It could be as long as 30 different principles. But the top five are what matter the most. These are known as your core values and anything that threatens them will send you into a tailspin. These core values define who you are as a person, so it is hard to go against them without causing a lot of internal upset. And if you're struggling with your mental health, some area of your life may be challenging one of those values. Knowing what they are is a good place to start when figuring out what is wrong.

DEFINE YOUR VALUES

With all that in mind, how do we value-audit our life?

Step 1: Check out the Value Audit list on page 232 and write down each of the values that you feel resonate with you. You don't have decide between any of them that feel similar right now. Just write them all down. Make sure you select at least ten.

Step 2: Think about how your life would feel *without* each particular value. Rate your feelings on a scale of one for 'I'd get by' and five for 'I'd be miserable'. For example, if honesty is one of the most important things to you, then having a liar in your life would make you miserable, so honesty would score five.

Step 3: Now order the list. The scores with the highest marks – those that would cause most misery if they were missing from your life – should rank highest on the list.

Step 4: Assessing this ranked list, is there anything that you'd swap around in order of importance? Anything that feels nuanced and slightly more or less important than its current standing? Make the swap.

Step 5: Focus on the top five. Write each down with its own heading, then underneath write out what that value means to you. For example, your top value might be financial stability. If so, then you'd write, 'Knowing I'm financially secure is the only way I know how to operate in the world,' or, 'When I'm not financially secure, my life feels chaotic.' Try and work with your *feelings* about each value. Write as much as you want here, because you'll get more out of the exercise the further you dig down into each value.

Step 6: Now, let's look at the different areas of your life. Use the Wheel of Life worksheet (see page 225) to audit how each area of your life is being affected. Aim to look at eight parts of your life. Areas you might want to include could be: Family, Finances, Home, Career, Fun, Friends, Personal Growth, Health, Spirituality, Travel, Love Life, Social Life, Community Life and so on.

Step 7: Assess each area of your life, by checking in with your core values. Is this area aligned to those values? Is there anything that's out of alignment? If so, what can I change in this area to better fit my values? Mark its alignment on a scale of zero to ten, with ten being fully aligned. You'll quickly see which area needs the most work first and can then tackle them in order.

Step 8: Once you know which areas need improvement, make a plan to change them one by one. Do not feel overwhelmed if there are a lot of changes on your list. Your life doesn't need to be perfect right now, this minute. Just *start*, then month by month you'll start to notice how different your life feels when you're living in alignment with your core values.

BUNDLE OF FLUFF

I haven't had the easiest few years and when my parents got a dog, Paddington, I realized just how much I needed one of my own. Paddington is a walking bundle of joy and Mum and Dad credit him with saving their lives after my brother died. How could I not want one for myself?

So, a year later, I got Rolo – a fluffy Cavapoo – who brings joy into my life on a daily basis. I can't think of a single thing in my life that brings me more happiness than this dog. His general enthusiasm for life is infectious and he has an ability to wipe loneliness from my life like nothing else. He's also a conversation starter when we're out for a walk, so even on days when I haven't met many people, his sheer presence means that I always have a few kind words from a stranger thrown my way, thanks to his devilish good looks.

I appreciate that Rolo is an extrinsic 'thing' outside of myself, but his presence aligns with my values. I love animals and believe they have a lot to teach us. And he does. I learn on a daily basis through him. I learn how fun life can be. I learn that it's possible to live as if someone left the gate open and charge into my day with excitement and vigour. I learn to rest when I need to. Rolo brings me happiness by teaching me what matters.

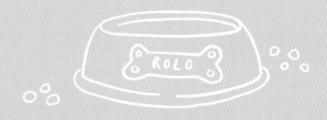

REACH OUT

Happy people show gratitude daily. Right now, is there someone in your life who you could thank with a quick text, call or note? If so, do it. They'll value your appreciation and you'll feel good for acknowledging it. It's like an instant hit of happy!

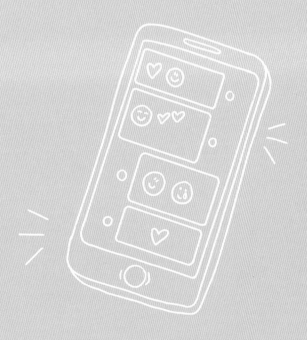

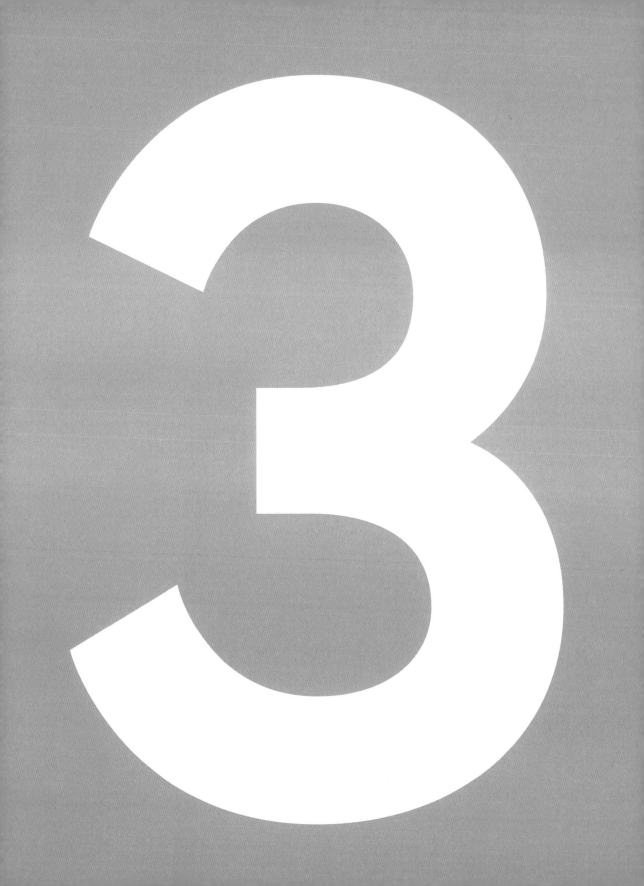

MENTAL
FITNESS
FOUNDATIONS

MAKE FOOD
YOUR FRIEND

What you eat will affect how you feel. Choose
to boost your mood with foods that support
your mental fitness, rather than fight it.

I often liken the human body to a sports car. It has amazing capabilities, but if you want peak performance, you need to look after it and that means filling it up with decent fuel. I don't think you need me to tell you that a balanced diet, such as the Mediterranean diet, is important for staying healthy, fighting off illness and generally keeping physically well. But you might not be aware of just how important nutrition is for your brain function, mental and emotional health, too.

FOOD IS NOT THE ENEMY

We live in a world that wants to make food a foe in some way. We're sold the idea that bodily aesthetics matter, regardless of cost, and that starving ourselves for beauty or status is somehow a necessary evil. Well, that's all lies. Food is not the enemy, in fact it's your friend. And it's time we all started to look at it that way.

I've seen patients come into the emergency department after collapsing or fainting because they've been dieting in an extreme way. I've seen people in my friendship groups follow faddy eating regimes and start to really struggle to function normally. When I lived on protein shakes prior to my *Love Island* appearance, I felt pretty miserable. Cutting out real food and food groups is no way to treat your body and mind. It's going to affect your mood – and not in a good way.

Severely restricting your calorie intake is a no-no, because your brain is greedy for energy; it uses about 20 per cent of your daily calories just to keep you ticking over. If you want to maintain good concentration and focus during the day, feed your mind.

Forget low- or no-fat, because a significant proportion of your brain is made from fat and therefore needs an intake of healthy fats to function well. While it doesn't use fats as an energy source, it does use omega-3 fatty acids to build and repair brain cells. Studies have linked omega-3 intake to better blood flow to the brain as well as improved cognition (thinking ability).[19]

And forget low- or no-carb, because your brain's preferred energy source is the glucose your body makes when it breaks down the carbohydrates you eat. Yes, it can survive on ketones – substances made by your liver when carbohydrates are in short supply (such as when you're on a low-carb keto diet) – but it's not optimal and I wouldn't recommend it. Bear in mind, too, that fruit and vegetables are carbohydrates, as well as sources of the antioxidants our brains need to stave off the ageing process.

Food is there to fuel us, power us, repair us. If we miss out on any part of that chain, we risk our health. A balanced eating plan will keep you looking and feeling your best. It will help you turn food back into a friend, a friend you dine with. And it will do your brain the world of good in the process too.

PLAN WHAT TO EAT

If I'm eating well, choosing healthy unprocessed food, a rainbow of fruit and veg every day and cooking for myself as much as I can, I definitely feel better for it. You know what it's like when you have a few bad days of eating. Allergies and intolerances flare up, energy and concentration are poor and you just feel terrible. It's when we're busiest and most stressed that we most need to eat well, and, at those times, it's unfortunately another aspect of self-care that tends to go out of the window. But these days, eating well to pre-empt stressful times is something I've learned to prioritize.

My work offers something different every day – whether that be a new location or a late finish – and if I'm not careful, I can lean too heavily on food delivery apps when I get back home too late to drop by the market. I've learned to think and plan ahead as much as I can. For example, when I'm on my feet all day, I need to have a good meal and carry healthy snacks with me. Otherwise, I'll just grab whatever I can find for an energy boost, usually less-than-healthy stuff because it's quick and easy. I try to batch-cook, making extra at an evening meal so I have leftovers for lunch. And I stock up on healthy snacks, such as nuts, to keep in my bag.

Staying hydrated is always important, but especially when we're busy and need to focus. It's a basic, but something a lot of people neglect. We humans consist of up to 60 per cent water, while the brain itself is 80–85 per cent water.[20] What happens if you go all day without drinking? Surprise surprise, you'll feel worse for it. I'd recommend having a refillable bottle of pure water (tap water is fine), so you can monitor your intake. Fizzy drinks and caffeine don't count, as they have the opposite effect of dehydrating you, so keep them to a minimum.

And on the subject of caffeine, really try not to rely on it to give you energy all the time. I've been there. You just end up with crashes in between coffees. People are susceptible to caffeine in different amounts, but if you suffer from anxiety and stress, I'd urge you to cut right down. It does make you jittery and it's not a reliable source of energy. I do enjoy a coffee, but I stick to mornings only and often I'll have decaf anyhow. It's made such a difference to how I feel.

WHAT'S YOUR GUT REACTION?

It might surprise you to learn that there's a connection between your gut and your brain. It shouldn't, though, if you think about all the phrases we use, such as 'gut-wrenching', 'gut instinct', 'gutted', not to mention 'butterflies in your tummy'. They all refer to the digestive system, but they're describing an emotional state: a feeling.

The link is literal, not just metaphorical, because our gut and brains are connected by the millions of nerves that make up the enteric nervous system, an enormous connection of neurons that deal specifically with gastrointestinal activity. This system communicates with your central nervous system and the communication is driven by your gut microbiome.

'Microbiome' is the name for the trillions of micro-organisms that naturally inhabit your digestive tract, microbes including bacteria, fungi, viruses and parasites, as well as all their genetic material and what they produce. As they help to digest your food they release chemical messengers, short-chain fatty acids, vitamins, enzymes and hormones that travel around your body, fulfilling various important – even essential – roles. A healthy, abundant and diverse microbiome is linked not just with better digestion but with better immunity and overall health, too. And we can encourage that diversity through our food choices.

Research is still very much in the early stages, but associations have been made between a disrupted microbiome (dysbiosis) and stress, depression and anxiety, as well as with irritable bowel syndrome (IBS). Scientists can't yet be sure whether depression results in an imbalance through poor food choices, or whether it works the other way around, but the state of your microbiome can actually lead to mental illness. Add to this the fact that everyone's microbiome is unique, like a fingerprint, and it's certainly not yet possible to treat these conditions with a one size-fits-all plan. But, by following a healthy, balanced diet, we're more likely to feel good. And one of the biggest lessons that dietitians tell us is that gut microbes feast on fibre.

Fibre might seem like such a simple solution, but, if you glance over any of the nutritional counts on the packages of the food you're eating, you'll find that very few include large amounts of fibre. Most adults are only eating 20 g (¾ oz) a day, when we should be eating at least 30 g (1 oz). Fibre helps with digestion and the release of toxins from our bodies and having low levels of it will adversely affect both your gut and your mood. There's also strong evidence to suggest that eating plenty of fibre protects you from heart disease, stroke, type-2 diabetes and bowel cancer, so it's a no-brainer.

FOCUS ON FIBRE

Your gut microbiome needs an abundance of fibre-rich plant foods, which
is easy to achieve by eating plenty of vegetables and fruit (choose a
rainbow of colours for maximum diversity of nutrients), whole grains, beans
and pulses, nuts and seeds. You can also try including fermented foods
that are naturally probiotic, so that's things such as kefir (fermented milk),
natural 'live' yogurt, miso paste or soup, sauerkraut or kimchi (fermented
spicy greens) and kombucha (fizzy fermented tea).

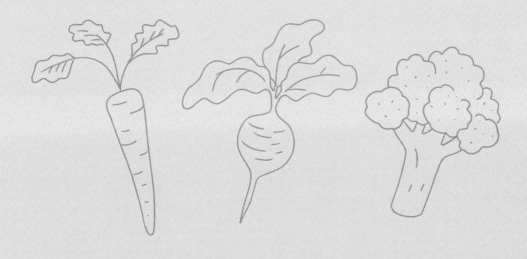

My body is not
TripAdvisor, so don't
leave a review.

IS BOOZE REALLY BAD NEWS?

Alcohol is troublesome for your mental health. It's not just the 'hangxiety' – that anxious feeling, or fear, you get with a hangover – it's the fact that regularly drinking will negatively affect your mood in the long term. Sometimes, when you can't put your finger on why you feel rubbish, the answer can be found in your booze consumption. If you're going out for a drink three or four nights a week – or if you're drinking at home every night – it's just not good news for your sleep, your mood, your hydration or your food choices. And that's without addressing how alcohol can make us behave, with implications for our relationships, or our safety itself through risk-taking.

Recently I have embraced a period of sobriety and I have swapped out alcoholic drinks with non-alcoholic alternatives. I'm not talking about having a juice or a lemonade: there's been a massive rise in the quality and quantity of 'adult' drinks, which I think is brilliant. It's the fastest-growing sector in the drinks market and you can find alcohol-free beers, ciders, wines, spirits and cocktails. Have a look around next time you're in the supermarket and you'll be surprised. You can even get lots of them in pubs and restaurants. Sobriety is very cool these days, as evidenced by the growth of Dry January, which 6.5 million people in the UK joined in January 2021, up from 3.9 million in January 2020.

So many people now are changing their relationship with alcohol, drinking less, not more. Overall consumption in the UK has fallen by 18 per cent since 2005, with the largest decreases seen for Gen Zs and Millennials.[21] I think this probably relates to greater awareness of how much it affects your mental health. Alcohol affects the chemical messengers in your brain. It suppresses certain neurotransmitters, giving you that feeling of inhibition, so you feel chattier and more confident, hence it can be attractive to those of us who have low mood. But the problem is, when you stop drinking, there's a rebound effect and you feel worse. I've had terrible anxiety, even verging on panic attacks, after drinking in the past. And it really messed with my sleep – one of the many reasons that I'm enjoying sobriety these days.

If you suspect your alcohol intake isn't helping your mental fitness, I'd really recommend cutting it down or out for a while. Try keeping a mood and sleep diary to see how it's helping. Or try out a tracking app, like the NHS's Drink Free Days. You'll also find lots of resources at the back of this book, including where to go if you're worried you have more serious issues with alcohol and need help: it's out there for you.

CALMING DOWN OUR RESPONSES

One of the latest theories about depression and other mental health conditions is that they could be rooted in inflammation. An inflammatory response is one of our body's natural defence mechanisms. Our tissues become inflamed in response to an injury, to protect them. Inflammation shows up in our bloodstream when we're fighting certain illnesses. It's a sign our immune system is doing what it's supposed to. But much like the fight-or-flight stress response (vital when we're in danger, harmful when it's switched on every day as in chronic stress), inflammation can occur when we *don't* want it to.

It's now accepted in the medical world that chronic, low-level inflammation is implicated in diabetes, heart disease, dementia and cancers. Targeting inflammatory or immune causes of these diseases has led to treatment breakthroughs, such as those for rheumatoid arthritis and other auto-immune conditions, as well as immunotherapy for some cancers. We also know that lifestyle factors such as a diet of ultra-processed foods (UPFs), obesity, being sedentary and stress all contribute to inflammation. And fortunately, these can be adjusted... if we choose.

Head of The University of Cambridge's department of psychiatry and author of *The Inflamed Mind*, Professor Edward Bullmore explains that doctors now realize the brain and body are more connected than previously thought and that inflammation could just as likely cause problems in the brain. He says it's 'beyond reasonable doubt' that depression and inflammation are linked. We're not yet certain which one causes the other. Yet studies have shown that if you deliberately cause an inflammatory response in the body, it causes inflammation in those parts of the brain associated with depression.[22]

What does this mean for us? Well, I'm sharing it here because it's a fascinating insight into what scientists are doing to try to improve our collective mental health. Could it be that, in the future, anti-inflammatory drugs will be used to prevent or control mental health conditions? Perhaps so, there's certainly much research being done right now in this very field.[23] What Prof Bullmore is clear about is that there are many combined causes of mental health conditions, so a single drug is never going to be the fix-all. Looking after your mental fitness means taking a 360° approach to your physical and emotional health.

On this subject, he also acknowledges there are many drug-free ways to help control inflammation, such as reducing stress, not smoking and – yes – improving your diet. Let's hope that science continues to speed ahead with findings in this exciting new area. But in the meantime, it can't hurt to make sure we're not promoting inflammation through our lifestyle.

HOW CAN FOOD HELP?

Nutritionists say it's mainly processed foods, red meat and alcohol that contribute to inflammation. So that means cutting down on fast food, ready-meals and all those pre-packaged foods with long ingredients labels that are so easy to eat. Foods that have been highly processed are usually pretty far from their natural state. They're likely to be high in sugar, unhealthy fats – such as saturated fat or manmade trans fats – and chemical additives. Think crisps and chips, desserts, cakes, pastries… I know, I know, some of the fun stuff. I think it helps to think of this food as deliberately designed to be tempting. Let's not allow the food manufacturers to win!

I'm not suggesting we should all be perfect, but an 80:20 approach is good. Aim to make healthy choices 80 per cent of the time, leaving 20 per cent for a more relaxed approach. I very much believe it's about finding what works for you and makes you feel good. That said, aiming to keep what you eat as natural as possible is a simple goal. Homemade is key.

Foods that are naturally anti-inflammatory are vegetables and fruits, whole grains, pulses, nuts and seeds, lean protein, healthy fats (particularly omega-3 essential fatty acids, found in oily fish, nuts and seeds) and many spices. You can probably see the similarities here with the foods recommended to best nourish your microbiome. And they're all packed with healthful nutrients such as vitamins, minerals and antioxidants.

This way of eating could also be described as a Mediterranean diet, widely acknowledged by doctors and dietitians worldwide to be healthy and promote longevity. A famous 2017 study called the SMILES Trial followed 67 volunteers with major depression over 12 weeks. It gave them either dietitian support and a Mediterranean-style eating plan, or social support. Those on the diet reported significantly greater improvements to their mood after 12 weeks than the control group. Although this is a small sample size, the study suggests that this sort of diet has a valuable place in the treatment of moderate to severe depression, and, I would add, for all of us.[24] There have been many more studies supporting such effects and there's even an emerging new field – nutritional psychiatry – so watch this space.

CHECK YOUR HEAD: BRAIN FOOD DOS

Fill up on…

Two litres (three
and a half pints) of
water a day.

Five portions of
fruit and veg as a
minimum.

Leafy or crunchy green
veg such as broccoli,
kale and spinach.

Antioxidant-rich
berries.

Nuts and
seeds.

Beans and
pulses.

Healthy fats (from
olive oil, avocados,
nuts and seeds).

Whole grain
(unprocessed)
carbohydrates.

Some lean meat
and fish (including
oily fish).

Spices such as turmeric,
chilli and ginger.

Soy products
such as tofu.

CHECK YOUR HEAD: BRAIN FOOD DON'TS

Cut down on...

Refined carbs (white bread, white rice, white pasta, baked goods).

Foods high in saturated or trans fats.

Foods with added sugar or salt.

Ultra-processed foods.

Caffeine.

Alcohol.

Red and processed meat

DON'T FORGET TO BREATHE

In moments of stress, we naturally tense our bodies and prepare for fight-or-flight. Make sure you've got some tools to remind you to drop your shoulders and relax.

One of the things that helps me best when I'm hit with a bout of anxiety is to describe objects in my line of sight, as I explained earlier with the simple trick of pouring – and drinking – a glass of water (see page 29). This is called the Five Senses Technique, and you can read more about it on page 162. It brings me right back to the moment and helps me realize that I'm not physically under threat. Over the years I have collected a range of techniques, including that one, which you can use in daily life to improve your mental fitness. You don't need to be a Zen Buddhist to keep calm in moments of crisis, some of the tools in my mental health toolkit (see pages 214–233) can help with just that. They're an easy and accessible way to reduce stress and boost your mood and brain function.

BE HERE NOW

One of the biggest wins for me and my mental health was finding something that brings me into the present moment. For me, that's walking. Without fail, I get out each morning for a brisk walk or 'stomp' for at least half an hour. It sets me up for the day and helps me approach whatever tasks I have lined up with a clearer head.

I've done this instinctively for many years and always thought of it as physical exercise, which of course it is. It gets my blood pumping and makes me feel energized. But more recently I've come to realize that, for me, these walks are as much for my mental as for my physical health, because they're mindful. When I'm walking, particularly out in nature, I'm not really dwelling over past events or projecting into the future. I'm taking in my surroundings, kicking leaves, breathing the fresh air – I'm using all my senses to be in the present. I'm connecting my body and mind.

That's what mindfulness is: being fully aware of your surroundings and thoughts in the here and now. And I think you can find it in many places. For you, it might be when you're running, listening to music, painting, cooking or gardening. It's usually something that requires some focus but not intense concentration.

You can do anything in a more mindful way. Have a go! Try eating an apple slowly while noticing its vibrant colour, hearing the crunch as you bite into it, smelling its sweet aroma, tasting its crisp tang and enjoying the juice and textures on your tongue. Noticing all these elements slows your brain down and brings you into the moment. You're not eating the apple mindlessly, while worrying about that email you have to send. Instead, you're spending five minutes focusing on the enjoyment of each bite. If you swap out mindlessness for mindfulness with as many tasks as possible – washing your hands, cooking your dinner, listening to music – then you'll punctuate your day with more moments of joy. You'll be completing the same tasks, but with the added bonus of relief from your worries. So switch your multi-tasking brain off for just a moment and enjoy.

If you want to actively cultivate a mindfulness practice, check out the resources section (see page 235) for some suggestions. And it's worth noting that the NHS actively recommends mindfulness as an intervention for depression and to improve mental wellbeing, so you could ask your GP about access to its resources.

I like this quote on the NHS website, from Professor Mark Williams, the former director of the Oxford Mindfulness Centre: 'It's easy to stop noticing the world around us. It's also easy to lose touch with the way our bodies are feeling and to end up "living in our heads" – caught up in our thoughts without stopping to notice how those thoughts are driving our emotions and behaviour. [Mindfulness] is about allowing ourselves to see the present moment clearly. When we do that, it can positively change the way we see ourselves and our lives.'

SIMPLIFYING MEDITATION

Meditation can sometimes seem rather difficult to master. But while there are many forms – some of which can be challenging – on the whole meditation is really just allowing yourself to be present to your thoughts, to observe them as you did your senses when you ate that apple.

Mindfulness is arguably one of the easiest ways into meditation, you could say it's the first step. If you practice mindfulness regularly, observing what is going on in the present moment, it will become easier to pick up a meditative practice that goes a level deeper to focus on your thoughts. You can find meditative practice in most religions.

The reasoning behind meditation is that, if we start to observe our thoughts as if they are transient objects in our head, we can see them as separate from us. Most of the time, when we're living through anxiety or depression, we can start to believe we *are* our thoughts. Meditation shows us that our thoughts are not *us*, but that they merely pass through like feelings. Once we start to observe our thoughts in this way, it quietens our racing minds. And sooner or later, with daily practice, we can get to a place where our thoughts are less intrusive and emotive. Now doesn't that sound promising?

There's a wealth of research supporting the effects of meditation on everything from long-term stress, through to blood pressure, memory and cognition, inflammation and pain, to anxiety. The science backs the centuries of use. There are also multiple forms of meditation available, so like everything else, try them and find a practice that works for you.

TYPES OF MEDITATION

Zen

This is probably what you visualize when someone uses the word 'meditation'. It is done sitting upright, following a breathing pattern, watching the belly rise and fall and allowing yourself to be fully present in the moment – to just be.

Transcendental

This is a more formal type and should be practiced twice a day for 20 minutes at a time. Your guide/facilitator will give you a mantra to repeat internally while practicing and that repetition is said to bring you to a state of peace.

Metta

Also known as Loving-Kindness meditation, this is a generous form in which you receive and send loving kindness to yourself, people you know and strangers. Most guides will suggest repeating a mantra verbally until you feel your compassion for yourself and others surpass your darker feelings.

Kundalini Yoga

This is a physically active form of meditation, where you're guided through movements, mantras and deep breathing by a teacher. Like other forms of yoga, it can also improve your physical strength and relieve muscular pain and stiffness.

COME UP FOR AIR

Learning to harness the power of your breath is an amazing tool for your mental wellness kit, so it's no surprise that 'breathwork' has become so popular in recent years. It's the formal practice of using breathing techniques for their physiological and psychological benefits. It's not rocket science, but it's definitely worth it.

I know, it sounds obvious: we all know how to breathe, right? But are you getting the most from this innate skill?

Stop right now. Let's try something.

Shut your eyes and listen to your breath. Take note of the count as you breathe in and out. Now, the next time you exhale, pause and notice how much slower that pace is, just because you're paying attention to it.

The next time you feel stressed or anxious, notice how you're breathing. It's highly likely to be fast and shallow; high in your chest rather than deep into your belly. Your pulse rate might be racing or you might have palpitations. You're in fight-or-flight mode for no good reason. The advice to 'take deep breaths' when you're super-stressed or nervous has a strong basis in science. And if you've ever done some breathing exercises at the end of a yoga class, say, you'll know what I mean – it brings you back into the present moment and relaxes you.

You don't have to look far for the research to back this up. Most breathing techniques are rooted in ancient traditions, so scientists are just confirming what people have known for millennia. Slowing your breathing down affects your central and autonomic nervous system, increasing heart rate variability. It changes brain activity, increasing alpha brainwaves and decreasing theta waves. All this has the effect of increasing oxygen exchange, slowing your heart rate and telling your brain you're safe and you're doing okay.

GETTING STARTED WITH BREATHWORK

A good place to start is simply noticing the sensation of your breath, then trying to lengthen and deepen it. You might recognize this as a mindfulness exercise too.

There are loads of different exercises you can do and I don't think any of them are necessarily better than the others, rather it's about finding what works for you and when. For example, you might find a focused breathing technique that helps you drift off to sleep, or one that makes you feel energized and alert.

There are countless books, YouTube videos and apps, as well as experts such as Wim Hof or James Nestor who offer guidance. Personally, I use breathwork to feel calmer in stressful situations – I've found it really useful during shifts on the emergency ward. And it's so useful for slowing me down when my anxiety levels are rising.

A good example was when I was supposed to be exchanging contracts on my apartment and the deal nearly fell through. At one point I was practically pulling my hair out from the stress. But I started simply counting my breaths to bring myself back to the moment. It worked.

It's a grounding technique and I do it before I give a talk or speech, too, as I find it focuses my mind. If I'm under pressure, I tend to catastrophize things. Counting my breaths for a few minutes helps to bring me back to the moment, so I can then focus on the task in front of me.

GROUND YOURSELF

Here are some exercises to try. You can do them standing, sitting, or wherever you're most comfortable. Nasal breathing is more efficient than breathing through your mouth, so whenever you remember, consciously shut your mouth. Be still, close your eyes if you can, before repeating the steps below.

Belly breathing
Breathe deeply so that your stomach is pushed out when your lungs are full and comes back in when you exhale. Notice the rise and fall of your belly.

Box breathing
Inhale for four counts, hold for four, exhale for four, hold for four.

Customize
Experiment with making your out-breath longer than your inhalation. Try breathing in for four, holding for seven, breathing out for eight. Repeat for a few minutes and see how you feel.

FIVE SENSES TECHNIQUE

When I'm in the middle of an intense bout of anxiety, I turn to the Five Senses Technique to really centre me. It begins with focusing on your breath, as I mentioned earlier. Take slow, long, deep breaths, placing a hand on your chest as you fill up your lungs. Then, following these steps, notice each of your senses:

Sight: Look around your immediate environment and name five things that you can see. Right now, for me, that's a glass, a pen, my phone, my laptop and my desk.

Touch: Next, walk around your immediate environment and touch four other things. For me, that's the solid floor beneath my feet, the leafy plant next to my desk, Rolo who's sleeping by my feet and the softness of my favourite T-shirt.

Sound: Now notice three things you can hear. For me, that's Rolo's snoring, the birds outside my window and the refrigerator's hum.

Smell: It's time to notice two things you can smell around you. For me, that's the candle in the room, also fresh-cut grass through my open window.

Taste: Finally, notice one thing you can taste. It's probably something you ate or drank earlier today. For me, it's eggs benedict. I love hollandaise sauce!

Once you've completed all these steps, you'll realize the issue that was causing so much distress has lost some of its power. And you are now more in the present and in control of how you feel.

SURROUND YOURSELF WITH PEACE

If you practiced that Five Senses Technique while reading the text, you'll have noticed your environment a lot, perhaps more than you did before. Sometimes we forget about our immediate surroundings because we have become so familiar with them, but that doesn't mean they're not affecting our mental health.

Whether we acknowledge it or not, the environment in which we live is seeping into our subconscious state.

A cluttered workspace can increase anxiety, the stressful commute we take can wear us down, the negative peer in our friendship group can lower our mood. It can all affect us, so we have to become more conscious of what – and who – we surround ourselves with.

To do that, it's time for an audit of your living environment. You need to know which parts of it are working for you and which are working against you. Once you know what to fix, you can go about doing something about it. But without that knowledge, you'll just suffer needlessly under unnecessary stresses.

Sometimes the most
productive thing
you can do is relax.

ENVIRONMENT 1: YOUR HOME

Whether you're living with your parents, your friends or alone, it's important to recognize what kind of stresses your home environment brings into your life. In fact, your home is the most important environment to keep healthy. After a long stressful day, or when a crisis hits, your home must feel like a haven, the security you feel at home will help you cope better in the world, which doesn't always feel within our control.

Action: Write out a heading for each room you use in your house. Under each heading, note what you use the room for, whether that's relaxing, sleeping, working or cooking. Some rooms may be multi-purpose, especially now that more of us are working from home. Note all those details. Now, list how you feel when you're in each room. This may seem like a silly request, but if you feel anxious in your bedroom (because it's now your home office too), you will get no sleep. If you feel stressed in your kitchen, then your meals will reflect his. Once you know the rooms that are bringing up negativity, brainstorm some ideas that can help to fix the situation. Can you declutter your kitchen cupboards to create a calmer space? Can you work at the kitchen table instead of your bedroom? Or, if you're sharing with flatmates who also work from home, could you swap rooms for the work part of the day, so nobody is taking their work into their own bedroom? The end goal is to create as much peace as possible. That may involve a plan to move somewhere else, to fit your needs. Whatever the result, aim to make home the best place it can be.

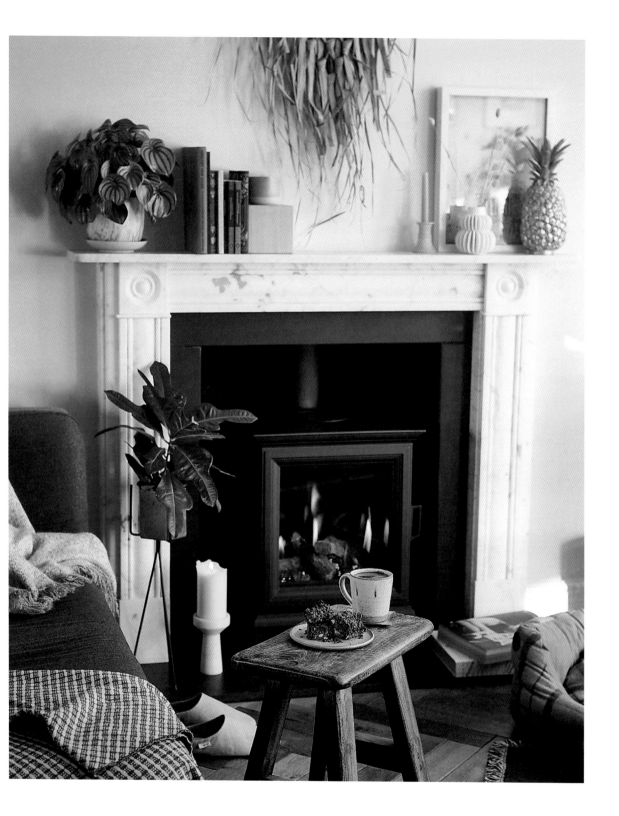

ENVIRONMENT 2: YOUR DAILY COMMUTE

Even though more of us are working from home than ever before, when we do venture out for our commute, a stressful ride can feel like a shock to the system. Living in London, I know this all too well. I cycle most places, but have noticed that I change my route based on the traffic. Of course, traffic doesn't really matter to a cyclist in terms of time, but in terms of stress, it does. A change in route can have huge benefits, as I found when I decided to cycle through Hyde Park, instead of through the car-packed streets. Is there a way you can rework your commute?

Action: Write out all the regular trips you take. That could include your commute to work, your drive to the supermarket, your train trip home to your parents' house. Now, as before, assess each trip, by asking yourself how you feel when you're taking them. If the answer is negative, brainstorm ways you can rework your routine. Could you walk some of the way to work? Through a park, perhaps? Could you buy your groceries online to avoid traffic and angry drivers? Could you plan to travel to see your parents on quiet weekends, rather than stressful public holidays?

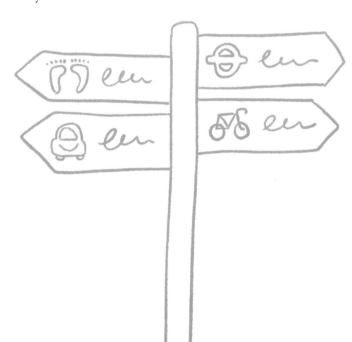

ENVIRONMENT 3: YOUR PEOPLE

As you know from the 'Connection is your superpower' chapter (see pages 46–57), loneliness is more detrimental to your health than smoking or obesity. But loneliness is not a lack of people, it's a lack of *connection*. You can be surrounded by people – who perhaps you even call friends – but feel incredibly isolated and misunderstood. This is loneliness and it is unhealthy. It's important to keep track of how you feel around the people you surround yourself with, and to make changes when necessary.

Action: Write out a list of all the people you interact with on a regular basis. This could include family, friends, colleagues, teammates, add anyone and everyone. Now, beside each person, note how you feel when you're around them, as well as why you think that is. For example, when you're around your best friend you might feel seen, heard, understood, because they always listen and reach out when you've been quiet for too long. Or, when you're around your boss, you could feel competent and motivated because they believe in your strengths. Or, when you're around your old school friend, you perhaps feel heavy, low and uninspired because they always complain about life.

Doing this audit, you'll quickly realize which relationships are lifting you up and which are pulling you down. Once you see this, try to spend more time with the former and less with the later.

Once you feel stronger, perhaps you can mend those negative relationships by talking to the person about how their behaviour makes you feel. We can often get into habitual dynamics in relationships, which can be changed once everyone is on the same page. Becoming aware of how your mood is affected by others will help you know who to go to in a crisis and who to avoid. And you may even realize that your ten college friends make you feel lonelier than your one work friend. In which case, choose quality over quantity every time!

You can assess any environment you find yourself in on a regular basis, whether that is the gym, the office or even your car. Just list out all the elements that matter and then figure out how you feel when you're in that space. Don't let familiarity cause stress, instead clean up your surroundings and help your mental health in the process.

GO OUTSIDE AND PLAY!

Leave the body aesthetics out of it. Make movement part of your daily routine and watch how your brain begins to thrive.

One of the easiest things you can do to boost your mood is to get your body moving... and yet it's sometimes also one of the hardest things. We can feel that we have to force ourselves to do any form of exercise. I believe that's because we've turned exercise into a competition, a race for perfection of some kind, something we have to do to *look* good rather than *feel* good.

Instead, we should look at exercise purely as movement and as personalized to your own taste as the food on your plate. It's up to you how you choose to move, just ensure you make the choice. Your brain – and body – will thank you for it.

MOTHER NATURE CAN HELP

Movement of any form is helpful when it comes to mental health. What's not often discussed is *where* we do that exercise. I aim to go to the gym three or four times a week, while also fitting in a run or a cycle. As we all know, life and work have a habit of getting in the way, so I'm relaxed about hitting those targets. If de-stressing is one of the goals of my exercise regime, then it seems pretty pointless getting stressed about it!

One thing that is non-negotiable for me is that daily 'stomp' I've mentioned before (see page 41). I don't count the steps or distance or anything like that, I just have a good walk. And I'm very strict about that because I think it's really, really important; if I miss it, I notice a huge difference in myself for the rest of the day. That's because, for me, it's not about the exercise per se. When it comes to going for a stomp, I find the effects on my mind to be absolutely transformative. What makes the difference to me is the fact of being outside, enjoying the fresh air and soaking up the natural world.

EXPLORE ECOTHERAPY

It's not just about enjoying the wind in your hair or the rain on your face, there are real tangible benefits to be had from being outside. The Royal Horticultural Society (RHS) carried out a study into nature and mental health and found that being in nature promotes calm by reducing anxiety, encouraging confidence, building a connection with your surroundings and creating a feeling of general ease.[25] We humans are not supposed to sit still in boxes all day, and it's so important to counteract our indoor screen-staring time with time spent outdoors, being active in nature.

Studies have shown how just being among greenery is good for both mind and body. It's called ecotherapy, and the RHS study found gardening and tending to plants is therapeutic as well, because you're nurturing something and being responsible for it thriving.

If you, like me, live in an apartment in a big city, it may seem that green space is limited. But in my experience, pockets of green can always be found, we just have to seek them out, which can be fun in itself and counts as even more time outdoors! Think local parks, a window box, a tree or a shrub, or even pavement weeds.

Research shows that just looking at green, natural scenes is good for our mental wellbeing. Ideally we should get outside into nature and exercise. But the next best thing is surrounding ourselves with as much nature as we can: plants, flowers, birds, butterflies.

I may not have a garden, but I have houseplants at home and it feels good to look after them and see them grow. They create a calming environment for me and, just as with my morning stomp, I feel the difference if I don't spend a few minutes a day tending to them. So do they!

If plants are too much hassle, or you don't have room, even just looking at pictures of nature can help de-stress us.[26] Having a screensaver that's a beautiful natural image of a waterfall or rainforest will send calming signals to your brain. That is because we're hardwired to respond positively to fractals – natural patterns found in clouds, snowflakes, raindrops, streams, lakes and trees – with one study finding exposure to them can help us reduce stress 60 per cent quicker.[27] Even looking at fractals for a short amount of time gives us a spike in alpha brainwaves and activates the area of the brain that helps us regulate emotion.

ACTIVISM EASES ANXIETY

As we watch the natural environment around us change year-on-year, it's not surprising that some of us are becoming increasingly mentally affected by the climate crisis. The Royal College of Psychiatry posted about the link between mental illness and climate change in 2021.[28] It found that 84 per cent of the UK public think that in a decade's time, the climate and ecological emergencies will affect mental health at least as much as unemployment; 60 per cent believe that these ecological emergencies are affecting their mental health now.

We all have a deep level of unease about the destruction of nature. I think spending more time in nature and getting involved, engaging and doing what we can for the environment can be helpful on all sorts of levels: for the planet, for each other and for ourselves. If you feel the need to take action yourself, then look for community initiatives that can help in some small way. Taking proactive steps will help relieve some of the anxiety that it's causing in the interim.

THE BIOLOGY OF MOVEMENT

If I see a patient who has depression, I'll always suggest exercise. Indeed, it's now recommended by the National Institute for Health and Care Excellence (NICE). Doctors can prescribe exercise for a range of conditions, including depression. Prescriptions usually take the form of advising three to four sessions of 45–60 minutes each week, and healthcare professionals can provide access to groups or classes to help you.[29]

Even in severe cases, where people are on multiple therapies, I'll take a multi-faceted approach that includes lifestyle changes including exercise. I'm not saying exercise alone is a cure-all, but it can definitely play a big part in prevention and relief. If done in combination with healthy eating, stress reduction and staying socially connected – as well as talking therapies and medication, if needed – then it's going to make a big difference.

The psychological and physical benefits of exercise undoubtably improve mood and anxiety.[30] Why is this? On a biological level, we know exercise gets your heart rate up, your blood pumping and oxygen flowing. But it also releases endorphins – the body's natural feelgood chemicals – into your bloodstream, while decreasing stress hormones such as cortisol. Even as little as 30 minutes a day can make a massive difference. Plus, exercise helps promote the growth of new neurons in key areas of the brain including the hippocampus, which recent research has found may influence conditions such as addiction, anxiety and depression.[31]

But what's going on with exercise and mood on a psychological level? I think a huge part of it is confidence. It really builds your self-esteem just getting out there and doing something and that only increases as you become more competent. Then there's the mindfulness: you're much more present in the moment, especially when you're working hard. Exercising also gives us something to focus on outside of our worries and anxieties and can even offer us the opportunity to process them at the same time. While not directly treating the causes of anxiety, getting outside and moving is a healthier coping strategy than dwelling on how we feel, or trying to distract ourselves with alcohol and/or food.

Active pursuits can create opportunities for social interaction, too, further enhancing your self-esteem and self-confidence. Then there's a sense of reward afterwards, that dopamine hit. You feel a sense of achievement that you've done something good for yourself – and you deserve it.

The most important relationship you will ever have is the one you have with yourself.

HOW TO MAKE THE FIRST STEP

I know this sounds simple on paper, but when you're feeling low,
sometimes even the prospect of going for a walk can feel like an
enormous mountain to conquer. That's when 'habit stacking'
can come in handy.

If you add your daily burst of exercise to something you already do,
then you're more likely to do it. What if every morning, while brushing
your teeth, you listened to your favourite song and danced around the
bathroom. Or try adding something you love to the process, such as
listening to your favourite podcast, like Stompcast (#shamelessplug)
while you walk or run every day. Just adding something you enjoy will
soften your resistance and help get you out of the door faster.

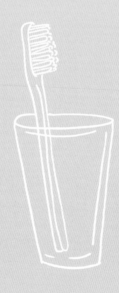

MIX IT UP TO STAY MOTIVATED

There are plenty of strategies to help with motivation, but in my opinion the most important is to choose a form of exercise you enjoy. If you hate running then don't make that your go-to exercise, because you simply won't do it. If you find something you like, it's much easier to stick to. And think outside the aerobic-exercise box: yoga and tai chi are relatively low-impact, but definitely count as exercise.

My second tip is to try and include a social element; exercising with friends is more fun, more motivating and makes you accountable. You have to show up if there's someone waiting for you. And, of course, those social connections can help with low mood, too. Instead of meeting friends at the pub or café, why not suggest a walk instead, or go dancing?

Virtually all the early support hubs I've visited around the UK include exercise as part of their schemes, partnering with local fitness initiatives or having visiting trainers. Blossom House in Liverpool, for example, offers boxercise and boxing coaching. Whatever the discipline, even if you've never tried it before, it's never too late to give it a go. Pick something new, join a friend at their chosen sport or activity, you never know what you might like unless you try it.

When filming the documentary *Our Young Mental Health Crisis*, I met a group of children who were really benefitting from something called surf therapy. Organised by The Wave Project initiative, children struggling with their mental health are taken to the coast and taught how to surf. Therapy like this has a dual purpose: not only is it getting children moving and exercising, but it's also doing so outside, helping them interact with nature. The kids told me how it had transformed their lives and I'm not surprised!

GET YOUR SWEAT ON!

Stumped for exercise ideas? Try one of these!

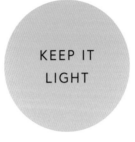

KEEP IT LIGHT

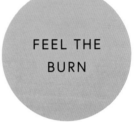

FEEL THE BURN

Learn to paddle board.

Bounce it out on
a mini trampoline.

Head out for a hike.

Try kickboxing.

Take your old roller-skates
out for a spin.

Join a dance class.

Flow through a yoga
session in the garden.

Go rock climbing.

Play frisbee in the park.

Hit the courts for
a game of tennis.

Brave the cold for a sea swim.

Sign up to a running club.

COLD COMFORT

You've probably noticed all the wild swimmers taking to our lakes, rivers and seas of late, and if you're not one of them, you may have questioned their sanity! Sure, you can understand the need to cool down with a dip in the warmer months, but why have so many people fallen in love with the Wim Hof way of doing things, diving into chilly waters in the winter?

The answer is endorphins. Cold-water swimming activates the pain-relieving chemical in order to deal with the sensation of the cold against our skin. That's why, after a few minutes, we no longer feel the temperature. Our body has neutralized the feeling of pain and the endorphins are giving us the natural high of enjoying the experience. Wild swimming is actually using the body's natural instincts to benefit us, rather than take us into fight-and-flight, as anxiety does. Cold-water swimming also boosts our immune system and improves our circulation, clarity and our libido, never mind the social benefits of meeting new mates before breakfast. Swim-win!

DON'T BEAT YOURSELF UP

Of course, there have been times in my life when I've struggled to exercise. I'm in that situation now, while I'm writing this, torn between going out to be active or finishing off this chapter! We all get busy and, when there's so much going on, our usual routine slips. If that happens, please don't be hard on yourself. And try not to have the mindset that returning to your routine means starting all over again. It doesn't, you have *not* lost the benefits of the activity you've done in the past, it doesn't work like that.

Every single time you exercise, you reap the benefits mentally and physically and you *don't* lose those benefits simply because you don't make it to the gym for a couple of weeks. Don't use a lapse as an excuse to stay away even longer. Just get back on it and you'll be surprised at how fit you still are. If you are exercising to keep your mental fitness up, then you never lose the benefits of a single session.

SELF-CARE ISN'T SELFISH

We need to break free from this belief that self-care is somehow selfish. That if you take time out to exercise (or do anything else to support your mental or physical fitness), you're cutting into time that should be spent working, or running errands, or being with your family. The fact is it's not just you who benefits when you make time for movement. Everyone and everything around you does, too.

For a start, your work improves because you're more energized, alert and productive. If you've got a difficult project coming up, it really pays to do some exercise beforehand, as you'll find it improves your clarity. When I was facing a revision session at university, I'd go to the gym first; I found that, when I came back, I was hyper-alert, calm and could concentrate much better. It's one of my favourite hacks.

In fact, being sedentary is bad for work in general, so I think it's better to divide your work up into short batches and make time for movement in between. Don't stay static, walk around when you're on the phone, or pop out to get a drink. You'll get more done in the long run.

And your relationships will improve along with your mood, so time you spend with loved ones will be of better quality. You're more likely to make better food and sleep choices, because you feel better about yourself. And you'll sleep better, which as we know is so important for mental wellbeing.

What I'm saying is, taking time out to exercise actually *gives* you more time for the rest of your life – and everyone else in it. So now that you've reached the end of this chapter, why not join me in taking a break, getting outside and getting active? I will if you will!

HACKS FOR ADDING MORE MOVEMENT TO YOUR LIFE:

1 If you have a meeting scheduled, make it a walking one.

2 Take the stairs whenever you can.

3 Walk a friend's dog, or join a dog-walking app.

4 If you WFH, walk a 30-minute loop as if commuting to work.

5 Play music while you cook or clean, it'll make you move naturally.

6 Get off public transport a stop early and walk the rest of the way.

7 Park further away than you need from your destination.

8 Try out a standing desk at the office.

9 Use a Pilates ball as your office chair.

10 During commercial breaks (or between streaming episodes),
stick on your favourite song and dance around your living room.

IT'S GOOD TO TALK

You don't have to rely on loved ones when you need to get your troubles off your chest. By visiting a therapist, you'll release the worries and learn how to cope better in future.

You know how useful it can be to talk through your problems with a good friend. They will listen, offer you support and check in on you to make sure everything is okay. But there are times when you can't reach out to a friend. Sometimes the problems we are dealing with feel insurmountable and too heavy for a friend to handle. Perhaps you don't want to burden them. Perhaps you don't want to worry loved ones with thoughts or feelings that you're not sure they'll understand. Perhaps you know that what you're going through needs some professional guidance.

That's where talking therapies can really help. Think of them as part of your mental fitness toolkit; something you can choose to access to maintain a healthy mind, prevent problems and process day-to-day stress, as well as to use in times of crisis. Talking therapies are a wonderful way of untangling the knots we create in our thinking. They can help us to reframe situations and better manage how we approach our life and the people in it.

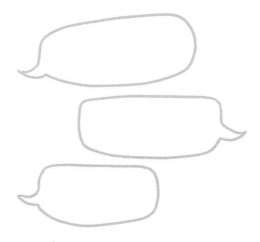

THERAPY IS FOR EVERYONE. NO, REALLY!

If you're already thinking, 'Nope, not for me, thanks Alex,' then I'm guessing you've probably bumped up against some of the stigma that's out there around 'talking it out'. So many of us have heard that we should bottle up our problems, keep a stiff upper lip. And while that might have been the advice of the past, we can clearly see that it didn't work.

Talking to a professional about yourself for hours can seem like a self-indulgent thing to do. Perhaps you're thinking, 'My problems aren't that big or bad,' or, 'Other people have it worse.' All pain is relative, so please don't minimize what you're feeling. You will not be judged for anything you talk about; your therapist is there to help you make sense of it, no matter how big or small you have decided it is. In fact, that is one of the great benefits of working with a professional in this space: while well-meaning friends and family might judge you for your thoughts, a therapist never will.

Therapy can help you to get through difficult times, such as a relationship break-up, job loss, or losing a loved one. It can help you to manage past or current trauma, deal with difficult emotions, or cope better with depression, anxiety and other mental health conditions, as well as with stress, or long-term physical-health problems.

Unsurprisingly, there are people who see therapy as something they do when they're feeling mentally healthy, as 'maintenance', in the same way as you don't stop exercising as soon as you get fit. This is certainly a view I've come to take since I started it. Therapy can be a valuable form of self-knowledge and is definitely a good way to learn the tools that can optimize your mental wellbeing. Sometimes it's hard to seek help when you're in the midst of a crisis, but having therapy once you start to come out of it can help you to process what's gone on.

KNOW YOUR THERAPIST

There are so many types of professionals in this area, it's good to know what each one does.

Psychiatrists are medical doctors who have additionally qualified in psychiatry: the study of mental health problems and their diagnosis, management and prevention. This is the type of specialist you might be referred to with more serious mental illnesses, for a clinical diagnosis and treatment plan. While they tend to look at the biological reasons for mental illness, psychiatrists may also have trained in psychotherapy (see below), so can offer talking treatments for the social and environmental causes of your condition, too.

Psychologists aren't usually medically qualified and cannot prescribe medication, but they have studied psychology – how people think, act, react and interact – to degree level or more. They can diagnose certain conditions based on their observations, or refer you to other specialists for further testing or treatment. They're interested in the normal functioning of the mind, behaviour and people's underlying thoughts, feelings and motivations. There are lots of different branches of psychology, such as health psychology – which looks at such things as behaviour change – or counselling psychology, which uses counselling skills in a therapy setting.

Psychotherapists are mental health professionals who are trained to use different types of talking therapy to help individuals, families and groups overcome their problems. They tend to deal with stress, emotional difficulties, relationship issues and problematic habits. There are lots of different types of therapy, ranging from solutions-based interventions to more classic analysis of why feelings are occurring. Your therapist should be able to talk you through which they use, why and what it involves. Someone can train as a psychotherapist or counsellor without any other qualifications (it is an in-depth course over three to four years), or they may be a psychiatrist, psychologist or other mental health worker who has completed this training as an add-on to their services.

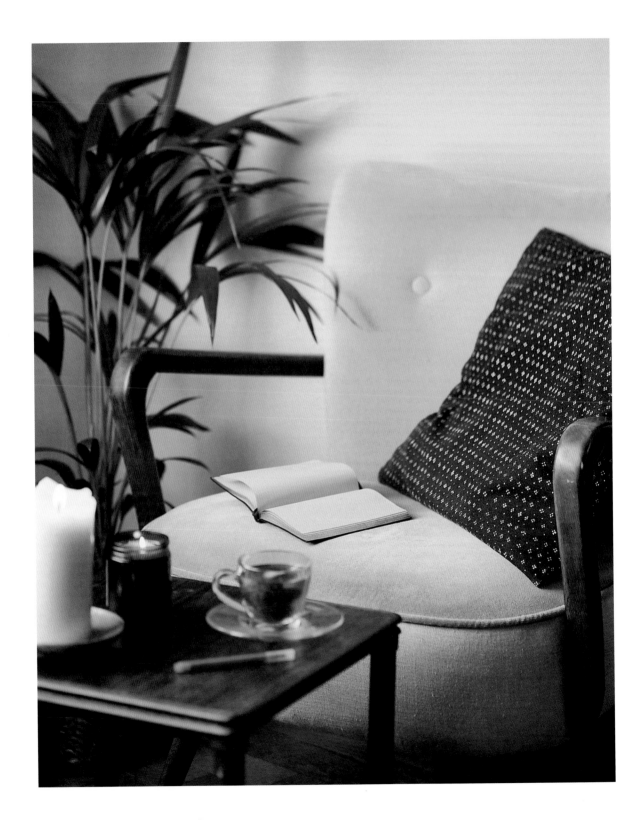

Counsellors are mental-health professionals who are trained in helping with immediate issues. You will often find counsellors operating within organizations, offering help when it is urgently needed. A counsellor will usually listen to you talking about your problems and prompt you with questions. They'll help you better understand yourself and find your own answers. Even though the title can be used colloquially to mean 'psychotherapist', counsellors do not dive into issues with the same level of depth that psychotherapists do. As with psychotherapy, someone can train to be a counsellor without previous qualifications (completing a three-year diploma course), or top up their existing knowledge within psychiatry, psychology or psychotherapy.

Life coach is an unprotected term, so anyone can use it to describe themselves, however qualified (or not) they may be. Life coaches tend to offer broader services around attaining personal and professional goals, such as careers, relationship or confidence coaching, rather than targeted mental health therapies. Many people with formal qualifications may also offer life-coaching services. And many life coaches *without* mental health qualifications may also get great results. But I would describe coaching as more of a maintenance service for when you're feeling okay and want to manage everyday stresses, rather than for treatment during a crisis.

BEWARE THE 'INSTA GURUS'

There's a large section of social media these days that's devoted to motivational messaging, life coaching, advice and support. Everything from those photos of sunsets overlaid with inspirational quotes to people documenting themselves pursuing healthy pursuits with #inspo to encourage you to do the same. Then, of course, there are trusted charities and organizations in the mental wellbeing sphere who offer ideas and suggestions. There are medical professionals sharing their knowledge, as well as real people sharing their experience. I like to think my social media offerings sit somewhere between the last two.

I am absolutely not opposed to social media being a source for good – I try incredibly hard to use my platform to help other people, and I do hope that I achieve that in some way. Positive movements can start when people get behind a hashtag, for example #BeKind, which followed the tragic death of UK TV star Caroline Flack. Or my own contribution in the form of #PostYourPill (see page 202), designed to remove the stigma around taking medication for mental illness.

What I want to caution against here is relying only on social media for your mental fitness. By all means take #inspo from that daily quote if it helps you. If there's a self-help professional whose feed you find motivating, go for it. But be aware that there are lots of charlatans out there, too. Anyone can call themselves an 'expert'. Don't sign your money away on e-books, courses or workshops without fully researching the providers.

Let social media be a handy resource for finding out more about where to go and what to do, as well as a support for whatever you're going through. But don't let it be all that you do.

WHERE TO START...

Depending on your situation, your doctor may refer you for therapy. It is often one of the first recommendations we make when faced with someone struggling with their mental health. That said, if you're in the UK, you can also refer yourself via the NHS Improving Access to Psychological Therapies (IAPT) service. Or you could speak to your company's HR department, as many employers now offer free and confidential external counselling services to staff.

However, if there is a long waiting list through the NHS or your employer, or you prefer to seek help privately, you can still ask your doctor for recommendations and to refer you. Practitioners may offer reduced rates if you're on a low income. Or you might be able to access services via one of the mental health charities (see page 235).

The British Association of Counsellors and Psychotherapists (BACP) is a reliable place to start if you're looking for private therapy and want to ensure your therapist or coach is registered. Likewise, the UK Council for Psychotherapy (UKCP) or the British Psychological Society (BPS) are other great organizations to use to check credentials (see page 235).

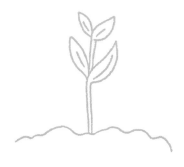

TYPES OF TALKING THERAPY

There are loads of different types of therapy and each therapist adds their own personality to the mix too, so it's worth shopping around to find what feels right for you – and don't give up at the first hurdle! Here are some of those you're most likely to come across:

COGNITIVE BEHAVIOURAL THERAPY

This can be a really effective treatment for lots of mental illnesses and it's widely available. Cognitive behavioural therapy (CBT) teaches you coping skills for situations that you find hard. Your psychotherapist will show you how your thoughts, beliefs and attitudes affect your feelings and actions. Put simply, CBT can get you out of negative thinking patterns, by showing you that you have a choice in how to react. It is considered a 'first-line' treatment, meaning you're likely to be offered CBT before other types of therapy or medication if you have mild to moderate symptoms.

You'll probably be offered a set number of sessions, as this isn't the type of therapy that carries on indefinitely. It's very practical and solutions-focused, which a lot of people like. You and your therapist might look together at things in your life you find hard, then examine how your negative thinking and behaviours are playing a role. You'll look at how you can challenge them and find an alternative. CBT sessions usually require a bit of homework too, such as keeping a diary, which is a really good habit to get into. That's the beauty of this approach: it's giving you a tool that you can use throughout life, long after your sessions have come to an end.

PSYCHOTHERAPY

There are many different types of therapy in which you talk through past experiences and explore your feelings. You might hear terms such as 'person-centred therapy', 'psychodynamic', 'Jungian therapy', or 'psychoanalysis'. What they all have in common is providing a safe space to talk with a trained professional who won't judge you. This can often be much easier than trying to talk with someone you know. Your therapist will help you look at reasons why you might feel the way you do, such as your subconscious mind or past experiences, then help you resolve your feelings, or learn to live with them. These sessions can be a good way to understand why you do the things you do and start to change – if that's what you want.

EYE MOVEMENT DESENSITIZING AND REPROCESSING

This is a treatment that has seen great results in patients with PTSD (see page 198); it's been shown to be really useful in dealing with symptoms arising from distressing memories and past experiences. In his documentary, *The Me You Can't See*, Prince Harry famously talked about using eye movement desensitizing and reprocessing (EMDR) to help deal with the trauma of losing his mother.

It works by putting you into a state similar to REM sleep (see page 62), which is a time when your brain is able to make new associations very quickly. EMDR taps into this high-speed processing and 'rewires' unresolved memories, so you don't feel them as acutely. Sessions combine talking therapy with side-to-side eye movements, which might sound strange, but it's done in an evidence-based, structured way to get results. These days it's used not just for PTSD but for depression, anxiety, addiction, behavioural issues and much more – some of which might be rooted in past trauma without you even knowing.

CLINICAL HYPNOTHERAPY

A branch of hypnotherapy that some people have found useful for dealing with mental ill health such as anxiety and panic attacks, OCD (see page 198), phobias, addictions, processing trauma and behaviour change. Singer Sam Smith grants his success with managing OCD to this form of therapy. A clinical hypnotherapist will talk through your issues, then lead you into a deeply relaxed state and talk to your subconscious mind to shift your thinking on these issues. The key is that you're in control at all times, so while you may feel like you're asleep and not remember the sessions, you don't have to take on any of the hypnotist's suggestions if you don't want to. Try to find one who has another healthcare qualification, such as psychology.

GROUP THERAPY

It might sound daunting to get together with strangers to talk about your problems, but this sort of support can be valuable, providing identification and sharing coping mechanisms. Group therapy sees one or more psychologists lead five to fifteen people in a session to heal issues around a shared pain. Groups are often organized around common issues, such as addiction, eating disorders, grief, social anxiety and so on. The sessions normally last an hour or two and are held weekly. Some people combine individual therapy with group sessions, while others just seek out group work.

These groups act as a healing community for people, in which they can see that they are not alone in the pain they are experiencing. Both talking and listening to others in this environment helps to create a sense of perspective about what you're going through. Groups also offer up a diversity of opinion, which widens the value that can be added. When someone else is seeing your situation through a totally different lens, it can help you to expand your own view and do the same.

ONLINE SERVICES

While online support services have long been available, the range and quality of what's on offer has really come into its own since the pandemic stopped much face-to-face therapy. They can provide a bridge between doctor visits and accessing in-person therapy when there's a waiting list. But they can also function well in their own right, for patients who maybe can't get to sessions in person, or who feel uncomfortable doing so. Online services these days can take the form of video calls, guided courses in practices such as mindfulness or CBT, and even in apps. There's some sound research to show they get results.

A good starting point for anyone waiting for talking therapies or wanting to find out more is the NHS Every Mind Matters platform (see page 235).

HELPLINES

There are so many incredible mental health charities, all listed in the Resources section (see page 235). Many have helplines you can call, whether you're in a crisis or you just need some practical advice. It's worth doing a little research when you're feeling good, finding some that really appeal to you, then saving their numbers in your phone. It's always better to be prepared…

PEER SUPPORT

This is like group therapy but without the therapist. Many charities and organizations have forums and private social media groups that allow you to chat with other people experiencing the same things as you. So many patients say to me it's that identification with others – the feeling of not being alone – that really helps them. Chatting to someone with first-hand experience of what you're going through can make a real difference to how you're feeling. As can knowing you're helping others, too.

It's not who you are that holds you back, it's who you think you're not.

FINDING THE RIGHT THERAPIST

I have weekly appointments with a psychotherapist and I find them really helpful. When busy-ness starts to overwhelm me, I know that my anxiety may start to rise. Talking to friends and family always helps, but sometimes you want to get all the small stuff (and often big stuff) off your chest without worrying you're taking up someone else's time. Telling someone who's paid to listen can feel easier.

What I have learned is that the time has to be right. Sometimes you're not in the right place to benefit, as was the case for me immediately after we lost Llŷr. Grief counselling was suggested to all of us, but for me I just wasn't ready to go there. It wouldn't have helped, because at that stage I wasn't able to be receptive to it. But now I'm in a better place and, since starting to deal with my anxiety, I've also felt more able to unpack some of the events of recent years.

My advice, if you're thinking about having some therapy, or if it's suggested to you, is to give it a go. Show up with an open mind and try not to be dismissive, even if you feel way out of your comfort zone – which you probably will, first time round. Commit to it. But also know that there's no one size-fits-all way to 'do' therapy.

And successful therapy can be a lot to do with the rapport you have with your therapist, so don't feel bad about changing them if the relationship doesn't feel right. I'm not seeing the same person now that I was originally. After about six sessions I didn't feel I was getting what I wanted, so I thanked them and said I'd be taking a break. I then sought out someone else who fitted my needs better and I haven't looked back. Remember you're not making a friend; you're using a professional service.

GETTING THE MOST FROM THERAPY

- **Shop around** – only use trusted sources (see page 235) and look at a therapist's qualifications and specialisms.

- **Find your fit** – ask for an initial chat or one-off session to see if you get a good feeling about a therapist. Ask questions about their approach, such as what therapy model they follow – Integrative, Psychoanalytical, Jungian and so on – and decide if that will work for you. If nothing else, ask them how a standard session would run, so you know what to expect.

- **Don't be afraid to press pause** – you should never feel pressured into having more appointments than you want or can afford. And it's fine to take a break.

- **If it's not working, change** – it might take you a few tries until you find someone you feel comfortable opening up to and that's okay. Any good therapist knows this and is not going to take it personally if you call time on the sessions. Trust me!

WHY MEDICAL HELP MATTERS

If you are feeling too low to manage the basics in life, visiting your doctor can help, as they will be able to offer a range of support to help get you back on track.

If you had a prolonged stomach illness, would you seek medical help? Probably, right? So why is it that so many people don't seek the same help when it comes to mental illness? Stigma has a lot to answer for on that front, and, while we are moving the dial slowly, each of us is responsible for our own mental health journey. And sometimes that involves talking to your doctor about what you're going through.

Visiting your GP about prolonged low mood or increasing anxiety is one of the healthiest steps you can take in managing your mental fitness. They are professionals who can help explain what you are experiencing from a medical perspective. Just as you would expect had you gone in with a stomach illness. This in itself can be reassuring, as it will shift your mindset from perhaps thinking that a decline in mental fitness is in some way a failure on your part, to regarding it as an illness, with symptoms of its own, that you need to recover from. Just like any other.

SYMPTOMS NOT STIGMA

When things have become really challenging, your first port of call should be your GP. Just as you would with any other part of your body, if you have a niggling concern about your mental health, then book yourself in for an appointment.

Your doctor will ask you a series of questions about how you've been feeling for the last two weeks (or longer). And from your answers, they will diagnose you, if appropriate. You may hear terms such as clinical depression or generalized anxiety disorder (see page 197), which are normally defined by the range of symptoms you've described and the length of time you've been feeling them.

What matters most right now is the treatment plan that your doctor devises to help you manage those symptoms. That plan will include elements we've discussed already – such as changes to your lifestyle or using talking therapies – but it may also include medication that can help lift you to a state where achieving those changes is more sustainable.

NAMING YOUR ILLNESS

After listening to you talk about your mental health, your GP will likely diagnose you with a specific mental illness, if it applies. They may point you towards the NHS website for more specific information on it, which can be helpful, but I find these definitions rarely offer the true experience of a condition. Here, I'm going to do my best to explain what each of these conditions *feels* like to live with, so you know when to seek help.

CLINICAL DEPRESSION

One of the most common misconceptions of depression is that is 'just' prolonged sadness. People say things like 'I'm depressed' when they're having an off day. But clinical depression is not about having the odd down day. Yes, people who are living with depression feel sadness, but it's more than that. It feels incapacitating for some. It sucks you dry of all joy; you no longer seek pleasure and you can't remember when you stopped or why. It starts to seep into your work life, where concentration becomes significantly harder. A job you once loved turns into a daily grind. Your self-esteem hits the floor and everything feels hopeless. You have zero energy for anything, your ability to sleep at night seems to have abandoned you. You can complete tasks, you can be a high-functioning adult, but behind the scenes you feel as if you're walking through treacle. A GP might diagnose you with clinical depression if you have been feeling symptoms on most days for two weeks or more.

Depending on how disruptive your symptoms are, they may diagnose you with mild, moderate or severe depression. It all comes down to how it uniquely feels for you. What I've just described to you is a sample of some of the things people feel when they're depressed. You may experience some of them, parts of them, all of them or none of them. For more information, head to the NHS website for guidance and advice on what to look out for.

GENERALIZED ANXIETY DISORDER

Much like depression, people can assume that those living with anxiety are just having a bout of nervousness. Of course, we all get anxious at times. If you've got a big presentation coming up, or an exam to sit, feeling anxious can actually produce clarity and focus. But generalized anxiety disorder (GAD) is not 'just' feeling nervous before a big event, it is feeling worried about life itself, all the time. You know that feeling after a big event, when you finally relax and every muscle in your body thanks you? Your shoulders drop, your breath deepens, you feel a sense of calm descend. Well, living with GAD means that this feeling rarely, if ever, arrives. You are alert, hypervigilant, always waiting for the next challenge. As soon as one anxious thought is resolved in your mind, another one appears. It's an endless stream of worry and fear. GAD is literally holding your body in a fight-or-flight response for far longer than it should be there. When our body thinks we're in danger like this, it releases stress hormones into our bloodstream. They activate our muscles, speed up our heart rate and prepare us for escape. If we were being chased through the streets of Cardiff by a lion, then we'd need this response to stay alive. When we're just reading an email at the bus stop, then we've been sent into overdrive. Living with anxiety can reduce the size of your life. It can make your existence small. You can start to avoid situations, people or places that may induce anxious thoughts. Instead of seeking joy, you solely seek safety, limiting where you go, what you do and with whom. You start to question everything that anyone says to you, doubting whether they like you, questioning their sincerity. Your trust in others declines, as you choose isolation over connection.

POST-TRAUMATIC STRESS DISORDER

Many of us have heard of post-traumatic stress disorder (PTSD) in relation to soldiers returning from war. As humans, we can try to understand how that experience could affect the psyche. But PTSD can happen to any of us, without living through a military conflict. The events that life throws at us can disrupt us in such a way that they leave a lasting impact. These can include experiencing or witnessing a natural disaster, a serious accident, a terrorist act, complicated childbirth, sexual violence or serious injury. That is not an exhaustive list, but all involve a trauma of some form, which PTSD prevents you from overcoming. When you are living with PTSD, your mind becomes a magnet for intrusive thoughts about the trauma, repeated involuntary memories, upsetting flashbacks or dreams. Your mind is trying

to replay the experience to make sense of it, but in doing so is retraumatizing you on a daily basis. When you can't trust your thoughts, this leads you to avoid people, places and situations that may trigger the memories. You'll then start to have distorted thoughts about yourself and others, as your mind tries to find a way to protect itself. Very quickly, someone who was an open, people-loving person can turn into a distrustful recluse. Added to this, the reactivity of your body will have changed. While you learn to understand what that means for you, you'll find yourself reacting to family and friends with angry outbursts or overly irritable behaviour. You become hypervigilant, get to a place where you trust no one – or very few people – and isolate yourself in your own mental prison for protection. PTSD can be extreme, but it doesn't take much for the mind to go into defence mode like this, so it's important to be aware of it as a possibility.

OBSESSIVE COMPULSIVE DISORDER

Obsessive compulsive disorder (OCD) can be crippling to those who live with it. It's made up of two parts, the obsessive side and the compulsive side. The obsessions are intrusive thoughts, worries or urges that repeatedly show up in your mind, regardless of what you're doing. Their presence is so persistent that it leads to anxiety. That's when the compulsions kick in. These are your mind's way of relieving that anxiety. For example, your obsessive thoughts could be around germs and cleanliness and your compulsion could be washing your hands for ten minutes. Compulsions can swallow up huge amounts of your day, which can lead you to avoid situations that might trigger them. For example, if you don't like germs, you might avoid taking public transport, meaning that you have to take a longer and/or more expensive route to work. They may stop you from going on nights out, as you find yourself stuck in a compulsion loop before you're due to leave the house. So it's not surprising that OCD dramatically affects relationships. As these obsessions and compulsions are not rational thoughts, partners, family and friends can find it hard to understand your actions. This will then lead to anxiety and doubts about your worth, sending you into an unhealthy self-esteem downwards spiral. You may feel ashamed of your behaviours and choose to isolate yourself, thus causing loneliness and potentially leading to depression. On top of this, the undercurrent of anxiety means that you're living in fear of your next trigger, never truly able to relax.

BIPOLAR DISORDER

As an outsider observing a family member or friend, bipolar disorder could be one of the most confusing conditions to understand. Although a potentially complex condition, its most defining characteristic is the exhibition of two very extreme and opposing states: mania and depression. When you are living through an episode of mania, you can feel immense joy and excitement. You are full of energy and bound through life with the greatest of ease. These are probably your most productive periods, when you clean your house from top to bottom before friends come over for a party. There is no limit to your energy when you are in this state. You become talkative to the point where others can't get a word in. You become impulsive and may feel reckless. Essentially, you're on the high of your life. Until you're not. One of the greatest dangers of mania is that you can put yourself and others at risk. When you're living through an episode of depression, which normally follows the mania, your mood does a handbrake turn. You'll exhibit most of the signs of depression (see page 197), but the fact that you just felt on top of the world makes this low feel heavier than ever. You may isolate yourself, afraid you'll scare people with your dramatic turnaround in mood. You may lose motivation, let the dishes pile up, find it hard to get out of bed and generally lose all interest in life. The time you spend in between these two states, not too high, not too low, is when you feel most yourself. You can get up, get things done, have everyday niggles or everyday joys, but all in all you feel balanced. You'll likely wish you could stay in this state for as long as possible.

Every person is different and their experience of bipolar disorder will vary. Some people will go between highs and lows rapidly, and others will find fluctuations in their mood to be less common. Some people may experience episodes when triggered by stress, others may find their time between episodes to be minimal. Your experience is all that matters when talking to your doctor. Tell them what *you* feel, don't worry about anyone else.

Be you.
Do you.
For you.

NO MORE SUFFERING IN SILENCE

Depending on your symptoms, and the degree of disruption they're causing to your life, your GP may suggest and prescribe medication. For many, this possibility is daunting, as it is laden with so much guilt and shame. Some are convinced that taking medication for a mental illness is a failure to 'adult'. That somehow we are at fault and that, if we avoid taking the medication, we will never have to admit that this is the case.

I hope, by this stage of the book, you have realized that mental illness is the result of the challenges life throws at us, coupled with a lack of knowledge about how to cope with them. In the same way that you wouldn't feel ashamed to have a sports injury, you shouldn't feel any shame for a mental illness – or for its treatment – especially given how many people are living with them.

According to the most recent statistics from Public Health England, an incredible 17 per cent of the adult population of England is taking antidepressants, that's 7.3 million people.[32] The number of prescriptions given out had almost doubled since 2008,[33] with similar trends seen in the rest of the UK and for teenagers, too.[34,35]

It won't surprise you to know that prescription rates have reached an all-time high since the pandemic of 2020.[36] The Office of National Statistics reported that rates of depression doubled during the crisis, with Gen Zs and Millennials most likely to be affected.[37] It's easy to see statistics like these as worrying, and newspaper headlines don't do much to help in that regard. They either suggest we're a nation of depressed people or that doctors are handing out meds too freely. And yes, there are issues with long waiting lists for therapy, with some people waiting months or even years to be seen. But I think there's a positive take, too. Could the flipside be that awareness around mental health is much higher, so fewer people are suffering in silence? And that, perhaps, doctors are taking patients' mental wellbeing more seriously?

I take an antidepressant for anxiety. For me, it has been life changing. I wish I'd tried it earlier and then I believe I would have coped better with a lot of experiences I've struggled with. But let's get things clear from the start: this chapter is not a sales pitch for antidepressants. I'm not suggesting you *should* take them, I'm simply saying you shouldn't discount them if they're needed.

While antidepressants worked for me, I wouldn't be doing my job as a doctor if I didn't stress that they aren't for everyone. Some people find no benefit in taking them at all, which is why it's important to keep track of how you feel while on your course, and to keep your doctor informed, so that other avenues can be explored if needed.

#POSTYOURPILL

Join the movement. When it comes to medication, you may find comfort in being part of a community: look up #postyourpill and read all the posts from others taking medication for their mental health. It started when I posted myself and my medication in November 2021, hoping to help release others from the stigma of taking antidepressants. Since then, it's taken on a life of its own. I no longer own it, but I love being part of it. On the first day of the month, we post a picture of our pill. If you're feeling brave, try it: you might find out others in your group are doing the same!

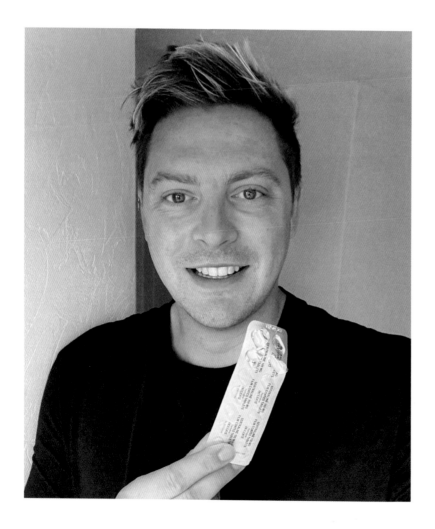

QUESTIONS TO ASK YOUR GP ABOUT MEDICATIONS

If you do decide that you'd like to take medication as part of your 360°
treatment plan, then I recommend informing yourself as much as possible.
Do your own research on any medications that you are prescribed, from
medical websites to other people's first-hand accounts of taking them. But
before you leave your doctor's office, here are some questions to ask, to support
that fact-gathering journey:

- **Why are you suggesting this medication?**

- **What specific condition are you treating me for?**

- **What do you think it can do for me?**

- **What are the alternatives?**

- **How long do you think I'll need to take it?**

- **How long will it take to work?**

- **What side effects do I need to be aware of?**

- **What do I do if I experience side effects I can't cope with?**

- **What should I do if I don't think they're working?**

- **How often will you check in with me?**

- **What else can I do to help myself?**

- **When will you review my response and dose?**

CONCLUSION

Let me ask you one more time.

How are you?

No, really. How are you?

This book has been a journey, for you and for me. I hope that, as we approach its end, you are feeling empowered. I hope you are feeling as though you are more in control of your mental health than ever before. I hope you realize where you're currently sitting on the mental health spectrum (see page 8). I hope you understand which areas of your life need a little work and feel grateful for those that don't. I hope you feel more grounded, and that you know where to look for stability, even if you were wobbling when you began reading. I hope this book has helped you take the first steps on your journey to finding peace.

I have wanted to write *The Mind Manual* for a long time. I wanted to create something that could help people with their mental health, whether they were floating or sinking, something that offered all the tools they needed to find balance, something they could return to again and again, to help buoy them, inform them, support them.

My own mental health journey has gone through so many twists and turns, even since I began writing this book. I am so grateful that I got to share it all with you. I find I can relate better to people who have been through similar trials to my own, and I hope sharing my own experiences has helped. I truly believe that, if you apply everything you learned in this book, you will find an inner resilience and self-confidence that can help you overcome anything.

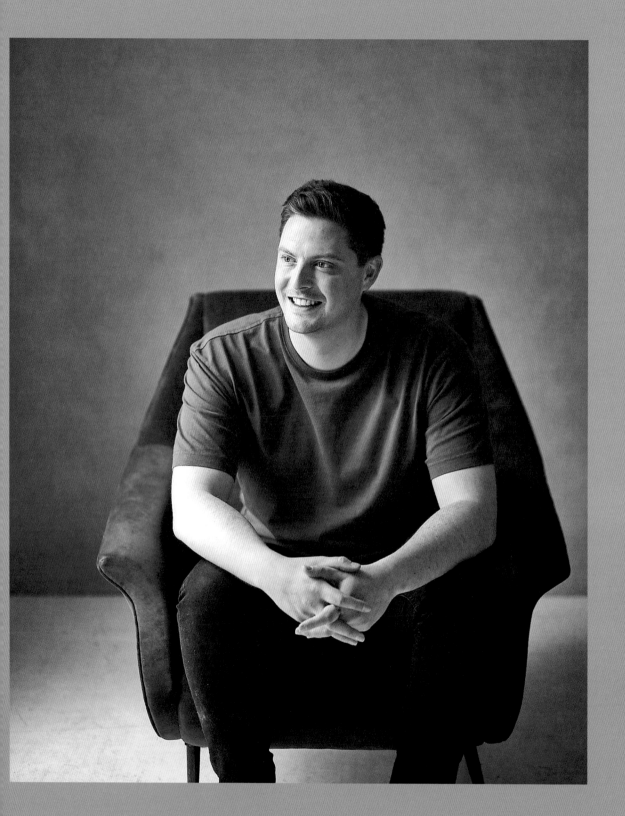

I still find life challenging at times. I have all the tools in this book at my disposal, but that doesn't mean I am perfect in applying them consistently. There are times when crisis hits and I forget to ground myself in the practices that I know work. At other times, although increasingly rarely, I even take my mental health for granted and slack off on doing the maintenance work for a while... until stress starts to creep up on me. What's different now, though, is that it doesn't take long before I realize that I'm not supporting myself. And when I do, I can quickly correct my course.

THE BALANCING ACT

When you apply mental fitness practices to your life on a daily basis, things change. When you check in on your baseline every few weeks, or audit each area of your life regularly, you'll start to become really familiar with how you feel. If someone asks, 'How are you?', you'll *know*. And that self-awareness is key to keeping your baseline balanced.

You now know that the end goal of a balanced mental baseline is not happiness, but peace. But what does a peaceful life look and feel like? The specifics will be different for everyone, but the best word to define it is 'harmony'. You feel like you're living in harmony with your values, your needs and desires. I'm not saying you won't have things that you'd like to improve, or that it's a destination in itself, but there will be an ease to life... most of the time. Aim for 80 per cent peace, not 100 per cent; we're dropping perfectionism, remember? With a ratio of 80:20, you'll find that you can handle anything that life throws at you, even if, as in recent years, it throws a lot. It may take years to reach this goal, but if you set your sights on it, you'll discover you operate from a place of self-compassion far more than you ever did before.

THE TRUTHS WE LIVE BY

Throughout these pages, you have learned how your mind can challenge you when it is not at its healthiest. In the same way a twisted ankle stops you from walking properly, mental illness stops you from thinking rationally. It can tell you lies, all under the guise of protection. But these lies, such as, 'Nobody cares what you're going through,' in fact make matters worse, isolating you from the very help you need. To help fight these untruths, we discovered seven truths that don't change, just because your brain does. If you haven't already, I'd recommend writing these down and displaying them somewhere prominent, so you can be reminded of them when you need them most. We've gone through each of them in depth in Part Two (see pages 42–139), but it's worth summarizing them here.

Our first truth is that **connection is your superpower**. Isolating yourself is one of the worst things you can do when you feel mentally ill, even though it is a go-to response for many of us. A better action is to seek connection. That is one of the fastest ways to combat the detrimental effects of loneliness. Having a sense of belonging and connection is paramount in supporting mental fitness. This is not a 'nice to have' item, it is imperative. Now that you know this, I hope you go out of your way to build connection in your life. If you don't have connection in your existing relationships, find volunteer groups to join. Establish a sense of community around yourself, so that you never feel like an outsider. *Take action on this*. It may come more naturally to some people, but it is definitely a challenge for others. If you're in the latter group, then put energy into building connections. Dedicate time to it. You won't regret it.

Our second truth is that **sleep will save you**. When you are struggling with a mental illness, such as depression, you may find yourself spending days in bed, napping your worries away. This creates a cycle of not sleeping at night, which leads to more day sleeping. It makes it harder and harder to pull yourself out of your depression. To break the cycle, you must start to think about your sleep hygiene and take action to clean it up. Even the smallest of steps can help. The world feels like a far kinder place after a good night's sleep, so seek it out. Take your sleep schedule seriously. If you try this for a few weeks and finally find yourself in a routine of sleeping for seven and a half hours each night, you'll be convinced of its importance just by noticing the difference in your coping abilities.

Our third truth is that **boundaries are beautiful**. In a world that tells us to do more, be more, work more, buy more, it can be hard to find the finish line. We may find we become 'yes people', pleasing others instead of ourselves and feeling resentful in the long run. Or worse, sending us into a state of physical or mental burnout. In order to establish healthy boundaries, both for ourselves and for those around us, we must learn to say 'no' regularly. We only have a limited amount of time on this earth and we should not be spending *any* of it doing those things we don't have the capacity or desire for. When you set boundaries – and stick to them – you free up yourself and your time for the things you really want. You add more satisfaction and joy to your life. And your relationships improve. It may seem counterintuitive to say that, but the happier you are with your choices, the more positivity you bring to the people in your life. And they feel it.

Our fourth truth is that **mistakes are a must-have**. Many of us are caught in a cycle of seeking perfectionism, while expecting to get there without making a single mistake. If that were a mathematical equation it would be unsolvable, as it is physically impossible to reach perfection, never mind getting there without making mistakes along the way. Mistakes are the stepping-stones to success and avoiding failure will mean living a very small life indeed. That's not what you want, is it? You don't want anxiety to set in, to stop you from living the life you want? Well then, you've got to make mistakes a must-have and watch yourself grow *even when you fail*.

Our fifth truth is that **stress is the enemy**. We all know this as fact. We know that stress kills. We've read all the news articles, blogs and memes. And yet, for some reason, we aren't listening. We're missing the point. Most of us live stressful lives, make stressful commutes, work stressful jobs, scroll stressful socials, book stressful holidays. For the most part, stress is an avoidable experience. You can make choices to sidestep it as much as possible. Sometimes this may mean making sacrifices, but if you weigh up the pros and cons, you'll find that stress is never the answer. The key to beating stress is in becoming very aware of its presence in your life. Where is it hiding in plain sight? And what can you do to release yourself from its grip? Whatever it is, do it, even if it takes years.

Our sixth truth is that **you are enough**. If there is one lie that depression and anxiety tell you more often than anything else, it is that 'You are not enough.' So, when you're seeking a foundation of robust mental health, it's good to audit your life, track down any feelings of impostor syndrome and eradicate as many as possible. All of us experience impostor syndrome in some shape or form, in some area of our lives. It is a universal human experience. Being aware of its presence is a good starting point for reducing its power. Once you find out where it's hiding in your life, use the Gather Evidence worksheet on page 222 to establish facts to fight it. You can learn to turn impostor syndrome into improver syndrome.

Our final truth is that **happiness is an inside job**. You would be forgiven for thinking otherwise, considering we live in a society that tells us that we can buy happiness with *stuff*. Small sparkly stuff, big noisy stuff, food stuff, clothes stuff, sport stuff, you name it, there's stuff for every unhappiness you feel. Right? Wrong. You now know this to be untrue. Happiness can only be found on the inside, and scientific research has found that those who feel a sense of belonging and give generously to others are happier than those who don't. It's the inner peace that those two factors provide that brings the happiness. So instead of wasting your money, invest in how you feel, not in what you own.

BUILD YOUR FOUNDATIONS

When you are living through a moment of crisis, you can feel as though the ground beneath you is unstable. Like you're wobbly on your feet, even if just theoretically. That's why it's so important to build mental fitness foundations. These will help to keep your footing secure, to allow you to feel supported even if chaos descends.

If you turn food into your friend, rather than your foe, you'll realize that it can do a lot to help your mental health. The right food choices, such as the Mediterranean diet, will nurture you, reducing inflammation and supporting your gut, in turn benefitting your mental health. If you're not in a position to overhaul your entire diet, aim for one meal at a time. Start with the one that's most challenging – if you grab something on the go for breakfast, say, or collapse with a takeaway in the evening – and aim to make it ten per cent healthier each day. This adds up quickly and you'll notice the benefits stacking up.

Anxiety can feel like your body is being squeezed in a vice. This comes from the muscular tension we experience from the shallow breathing and protective posturing. Establishing routines that combat the effects of this, such as breathwork and meditation, will keep your body balanced. And preparing yourself for challenges with the mindfulness tools in this book will support you during low moments, as well as help you to prevent them.

Our bodies are built for movement, but there is not a one-size-fits-all solution. Some of us love a good stomp, while others choose something more vigorous. We need to move away from the marketing spiel that exercise is purely for aesthetics, to make yourself 'look good'. In itself, this will add more stress to an already stressed body. Instead, we should use movement for mental clarity and calm. If you approach it in this way, you'll never fear it, but seek it out.

One of the most solid foundations you can offer your mental health is to create a support system around yourself. This can include family and friends, but at times, especially when we may need them the most, these may not be the people we want to burden with our worries. That's why a therapist is a great person to have within your support system. They are literally paid to listen to you, offer support and advice (depending on their qualifications) and can be a stable, constant voice across the years.

Finally, your mental fitness foundations should include visits to your doctor. Their medical help matters and can often release you from feeling as though mental difficulties are all your own fault. When a doctor sees something as medical/physical and explains it to you in those terms, it can instantly relieve us of the need to judge it. If you are prescribed medication to help, do your research, then go with what feels right for you. Don't let stigma stop you from getting your life back on track.

MENTAL HEALTH TOOLKIT

In the next part of this book (see pages 214–233), you will find a range of exercises and worksheets to complete. These will help you to build your mental health foundations, find your baseline, as well as support you when you feel challenged. Use them within the book, or buy yourself a journal to use for your mental fitness and complete them in that. The cognitive act of completing the exercises will often open up your awareness enough that action may not be required. But when it is, you know you have a guide with these tools. Exercises, such as the Wheel of Life (see page 225), can be repeated over and again throughout life, no matter where you're sitting on the mental health spectrum. I encourage you to spend time completing these over the next few weeks, as you start to establish new habits and mindsets. I find them fun.

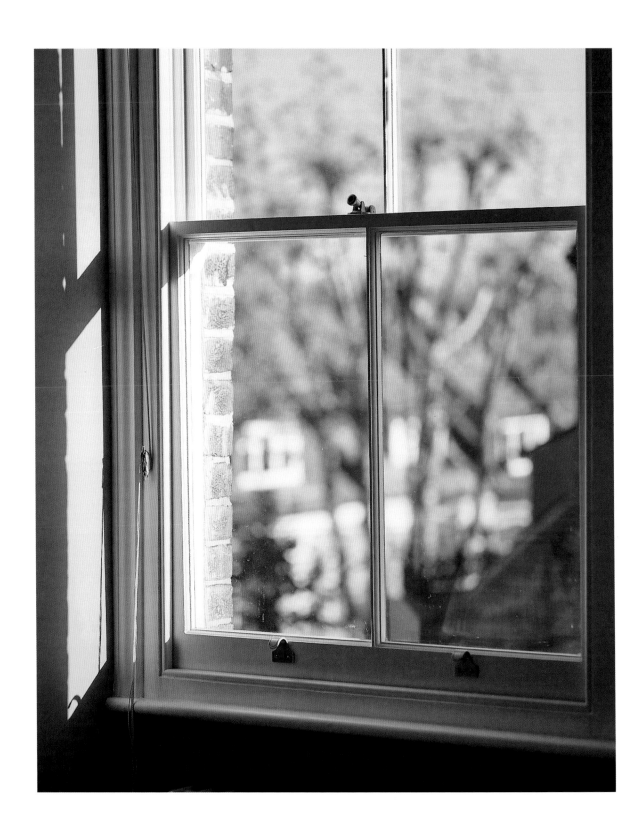

A PLACE TO BELONG

You are not alone in wanting to improve your mental fitness, there is a whole community of us out there. Join mental health communities online and you'll find many like-minded people who want to take care of themselves as best they can. They're not just interested in *looking* good, they want to *feel* good. They're making choices that reflect this desire. Sometimes these choices look like long periods of rest, sometimes they look like bursts of productivity, but all are made from an internal decision to be mentally fit. Come join us.

Together, we feel empowered to explore what mental health and fitness mean to us. We talk about it in safe spaces at first. We discuss it with friends and loved ones. And then, when we start to gain confidence and feel that our footing is secure, we venture out into the world. And we share our story and the tools we used to balance our baselines. We tell others how to find peace. We no longer let others suffer in silence, we speak up, we support, we all prosper.

I hope that the journey you are about to take brings harmony to your life.

I hope you come to love the choices that you make for yourself, as well as their positive effects on your health.

I hope you live with self-compassion and a little bit of grit.

I hope you spend your life learning and growing and sharing everything you know.

I hope you build a life of which you're really proud; one you never want to leave.

I hope you return to these pages often, and I hope that they help you find your inner peace.

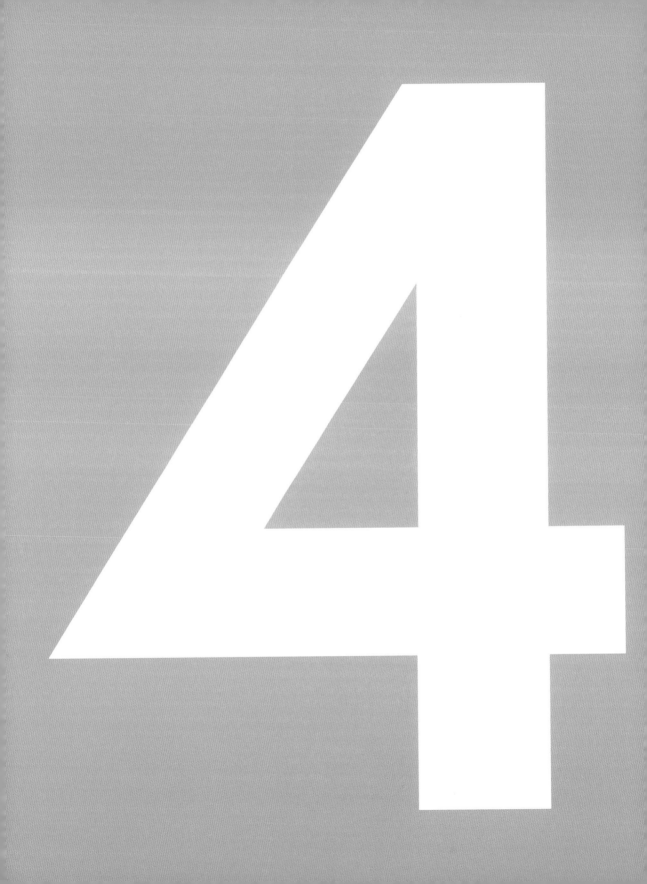

MENTAL
HEALTH
TOOLKIT

CREATE CONNECTION

Follow the guide below to design an action plan to use on those days when you feel lonely. Complete it when you're feeling good, so that you can offer yourself that energy on the days when you don't.

List each person you know who makes you feel you can be entirely yourself.

List your favourite local spots that make you feel connected to your community.

List the activities you love that make you feel vibrant and alive.

Make a date on your calendar to engage with at least one person/spot/activity from those lists every week. Or, for immediate action, add it to your day today.

GET GRATEFUL

Every evening before bed, make a gratitude list. This will help end the day with a sense of peace, even if some of it has been turbulent. Aim to list at least five things from your day that you are grateful for and why. You can include anything that made you feel blessed, big or small. You could be grateful for the pillow under your head, or the city you live in. Try to list five new things to write down every day, or, if you repeat something, to find a new reason why. This will encourage you to seek out the positive, even on the toughest days.

NORMALIZE 'NO'

Write down the five scenarios that come up in your life in which you most commonly end up saying 'yes' when you really mean to say 'no'. For example, you may always say 'yes' to overtime when you already have a full evening planned. Or you may want to avoid alcohol, but end up buckling when friends try to convince you to have a drink. Under each scenario, write out useful anchor phrases that you can use the next time you find yourself in this situation. Practice saying them in the mirror if that helps you feel more comfortable. And every time you use these anchor phrases, you'll feel a little stronger.

	SCENARIO	ANCHOR PHRASE
1		
2		
3		
4		
5		

DEAL WITH DOOM

When we are worried about something, we often consider a wide range of possible scenarios and how they could play out. Our brain tries to figure out how it would cope and worries about the possibility that it won't be able to. What you need to ask yourself is this: if the worst thing that could possibly happen did actually take place, how would you cope? Often, we discover that we would survive, that we would make the best of the bad situation and that we'd probably learn from it. The simple act of writing this out relieves your brain of the endless loop of possibilities. Those imagined doom-laden scenarios don't matter, because if you can survive the worst thing, then you can survive anything else too. Use the space below to unravel your doom forecasting.

What are you worried about?

What is the worst thing that could happen?

How would you cope?

What are you worried about?

What is the worst thing that could happen?

How would you cope?

What are you
worried about?

What is the worst thing
that could happen?

How would you cope?

What are you
worried about?

What is the worst thing
that could happen?

How would you cope?

What are you
worried about?

What is the worst thing
that could happen?

How would you cope?

WEAKEN WORRY

It's very easy to feel as though our problems are insurmountable and let them take up room in our life. One tool to help with this is to remember how much – or little – these same problems will matter in the future. You'll quickly realize that something that feels big is actually quite small in the grand scheme of things. Write out your worry below, then consider how important it will be at each of the marked moments in time.

- **What am I worried about?**
- **Will it matter in a year's time?**
- **Will it matter in five years' time?**
- **Will it matter in ten years' time?**
- **Will it matter in 100 years' time?**
- **Considering these answers, is it worth the energy I'm putting into it now?**

TALK THOUGHTS

Talking out our thoughts can be a useful way of unravelling them. Find yourself a thought buddy, someone whose opinion you trust and who is invested in your life as much as you are in theirs. It could be a family member or a very close friend. Then, every night if you need it, call each other for a quick chat about the thought of the day – the one thing that's been swirling round and round in your head and you haven't been able to release. Often, your brain is actually looking for an answer to the question this thought brings up, and talking it out with a thought buddy can help provide you with solutions.

You should both share your feelings on the call, so that it is connective on both sides. Not only will this ease a worried mind, but it will also bring you closer and allow you both to feel a sense of connection. When on the call, use the prompts below to help unravel the 'thought knot' in your head. It's also good to comment on how previous thoughts panned out; for example, how something that you discussed two weeks ago is no longer an issue at all. Learn from what that experience taught you, to understand how it can help future thought knots.

- **What is the thing I've been worrying most about today?**
- **What is my biggest fear with this issue?**
- **What is the worst-case scenario?**
- **How would I cope if that happened?**
- **What is an action I could take now to help relieve some pressure?**
- **What advice do you (thought buddy) have on this?**

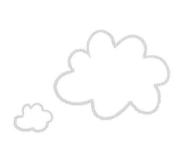

GATHER EVIDENCE

Impostor syndrome tells us that we're not good enough. It tries to convince us that we're going to get 'found out' and ostracized by others. To combat its powerful lies, get into the habit of gathering evidence to support the opposite. Your brain loves logic, so if you can provide evidence that a thought is untrue, it can't help but diminish its power. Use the tool below to question your intrusive thought and fight back with fact.

What is my impostor syndrome trying to convince me is true?

List four pieces of evidence to prove that this is a lie.

1

2

3

4

PREP YOUR PILL

In the first few weeks of taking antidepressants, you may find that your symptoms worsen. For that reason, it's good to create an action plan of how to access support during that period. Use the guide below to design a support structure for at least the first four weeks, and don't begin taking the medication until everything is in place.

- **Name at least one person (other than your doctor) who knows that you are starting antidepressants. You should inform them of how challenging it can be initially and get their permission to reach out 24/7 if things get bad.**
- **Research all the potential side effects of this specific drug. Create a list of side effects that you could handle on your own, and a list of side effects that you will need professional help to deal with.**

Handle on my own	Need help
1	1
2	2
3	3

List emergency contacts for times when you need professional help.

Doctor (including out of hours number):

Local support group (check out hubofhope.co.uk using your postcode):

Samaritans: 116 123

During the first four weeks, I will commit to completing each of the below daily.

Physical activity:

Connection activity:

Rest activity:

Journal activity:

TRACK YOUR MOOD

Even if you journal every day, it can be hard to figure out how you're feeling on the whole. Medical advice suggests that two or more weeks of low mood is cause for concern, but often we leave it far longer to reach out for help. The Traffic Light Technique is a great way to track your mood in general. Essentially, you use the colours of a traffic light to define how you feel on any given day. Green is positive, amber is middling and red is negative. Too many red days in a row would indicate that something is amiss. You can use this tool in your journal, at the dinner table with your family, or in a WhatsApp group with friends, to get an overall picture and catch a crisis before it happens.

Monday	○ ○ ○	Monday	○ ○ ○
Tuesday	○ ○ ○	Tuesday	○ ○ ○
Wednesday	○ ○ ○	Wednesday	○ ○ ○
Thursday	○ ○ ○	Thursday	○ ○ ○
Friday	○ ○ ○	Friday	○ ○ ○
Saturday	○ ○ ○	Saturday	○ ○ ○
Sunday	○ ○ ○	Sunday	○ ○ ○

Monday	○ ○ ○	Monday	○ ○ ○
Tuesday	○ ○ ○	Tuesday	○ ○ ○
Wednesday	○ ○ ○	Wednesday	○ ○ ○
Thursday	○ ○ ○	Thursday	○ ○ ○
Friday	○ ○ ○	Friday	○ ○ ○
Saturday	○ ○ ○	Saturday	○ ○ ○
Sunday	○ ○ ○	Sunday	○ ○ ○

Monday	○ ○ ○	Monday	○ ○ ○
Tuesday	○ ○ ○	Tuesday	○ ○ ○
Wednesday	○ ○ ○	Wednesday	○ ○ ○
Thursday	○ ○ ○	Thursday	○ ○ ○
Friday	○ ○ ○	Friday	○ ○ ○
Saturday	○ ○ ○	Saturday	○ ○ ○
Sunday	○ ○ ○	Sunday	○ ○ ○

AUDIT YOUR FEELINGS

The Wheel of Life is a coaching tool that has spread across multiple industries, because it is such a useful way to assess where our lives need improvement. Using the guide below, assess how satisfied you're feeling about each area you define within the wheel.

The centre of the circle indicates the least amount of satisfaction (scoring zero), and the outer edge of the circle indicates full satisfaction (scoring ten). You can use this wheel to audit any area of your life. If you can, try to fill out each area with a different colour. For example, if you've given one area a rating of six, colour in the area of the pie from the centre of the circle out to the six line. When completed, it will give you a visual overview of your feelings.

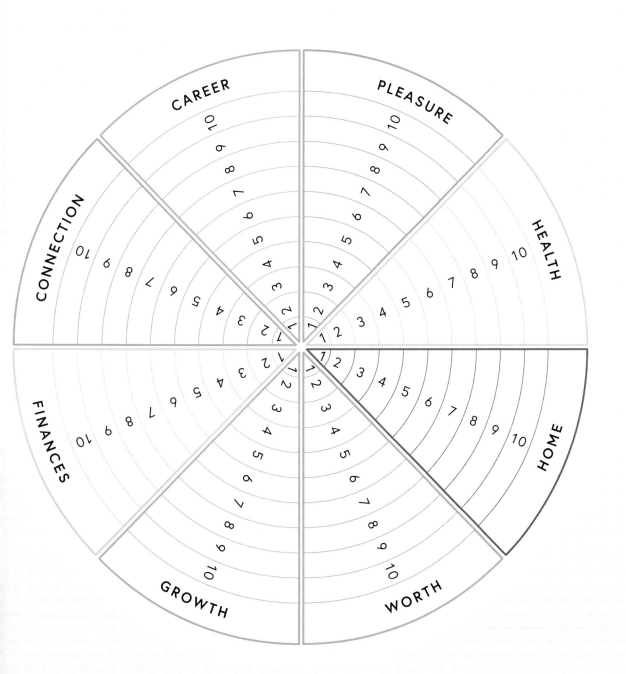

SPHERE OF INFLUENCE

Our brains often don't differentiate between worries. Everything can become an issue, with intrusive thoughts crowding in to clutter our mind. To kick yourself into a cognitive awakening, use this modified version of the Sphere of Influence. My best friend's dad taught me this when I was 14 and I've been using it ever since.

Draw a circle on a page. In the circle, write down all the worries you have that you have control over – that is to say, those that you can do something about. Outside the circle, put all the worries you have no control over. The simple action of doing that allows your brain to realize it can drop the heaviness of the worries outside the circle. They may have influence over your life, but you no longer need to worry about them. For the items within the circle, write out actions you can take to relieve the worry in some way. Try the Deal with Doom worst-case scenario worksheet, too (see page 220).

DUMP DUTIES

Sunday nights are traditionally filled with worry about the week ahead. We lie in bed hours after hitting the hay, thinking about all the things we need to do tomorrow, running through an open-ended to-do list… and we can find ourselves stuck in a loop.

To avoid this, get into the habit of dumping out your to-do list into a journal before bed. You can do this any and every night of the week, not just on Sundays. Once you've written your list, sign it, as a signal that you've committed to checking in on it in the morning. Tomorrow, over a hot drink first thing, you can decide what needs to be done and when. If you make this journaling part of your pre-sleep ritual, you'll find yourself nodding off faster than ever before.

VALUE AUDIT

Select all the qualities listed here that you feel resonate with how you view the world. Rate them in order. The top five are the priorities which define who you are as a person, also known as your core values. Consider how closely your life currently aligns to those qualities.

Acceptance	Being reasonable	Community	Determination	Expressive
Accomplishment	Being skilled	Compassion	Development	Fairness
Accountability	Being thoughtful	Competence	Devotion	Fame
Accuracy	Boldness	Concentration	Dignity	Family
Achievement	Bravery	Confidence	Discipline	Fidelity
Adaptability	Brilliance	Connection	Discovery	Focus
Alertness	Calm	Consistency	Drive	Foresight
Altruism	Candour	Contentment	Effectiveness	Fortitude
Ambition	Capable	Contribution	Efficiency	Freedom
Assertiveness	Careful	Control	Empathy	Friendship
Attentiveness	Certainty	Conviction	Empower	Fun
Awareness	Challenge	Cooperation	Endurance	Generosity
Balance	Charity	Courage	Energy	Genius
Beauty	Clarity	Courtesy	Enjoyment	Giving
Being admirable	Cleanliness	Creativity	Enthusiasm	Goodness
Being dynamic	Clever	Credibility	Equality	Grace
Being earnest	Comfort	Curiosity	Ethical	Gratitude
Being frank	Commitment	Decisiveness	Excellence	Greatness
Being methodical	Common sense	Dedication	Experience	Growth
Being personable	Communication	Dependability	Exploration	Happiness

Hard work	Lawful	Potential	Sensitivity	Teamwork
Harmony	Leadership	Power	Serenity	Temperance
Health	Learning	Present	Service	Thankful
Honesty	Liberty	Productivity	Sharing	Thorough
Honour	Logic	Professionalism	Significance	Thoughtful
Hope	Love	Prosperity	Silence	Tolerance
Humility	Loyalty	Purpose	Simplicity	Toughness
Imagination	Mastery	Quality	Sincerity	Tradition
Improvement	Maturity	Realistic	Skill	Tranquility
Independence	Meaning	Reason	Skillfulness	Transparency
Individuality	Moderation	Recognition	Smart	Trust
Innovation	Motivation	Recreation	Solitude	Truth
Inquisitive	Openness	Reflective	Spirituality	Understanding
Insightful	Optimism	Respect	Spontaneous	Uniqueness
Inspiring	Order	Responsibility	Stability	Unity
Integrity	Organization	Restraint	Status	Valour
Intelligence	Originality	Results-oriented	Stewardship	Vigour
Intensity	Passion	Reverence	Strength	Vision
Intuitive	Patience	Rigour	Structure	Vitality
Irreverent	Peace	Risk	Success	Wealth
Joy	Performance	Satisfaction	Support	Welcoming
Justice	Persistence	Security	Surprise	Winning
Kindness	Playfulness	Self-reliance	Sustainability	Wisdom
Knowledge	Poise	Selfless	Talent	Wonder

ENDNOTES

1 https://www.gov.uk/government/news/uk-flu-levels-according-to-phe-statistics-2019-to-2020

2 https://www2.deloitte.com/content/dam/Deloitte/global/Documents/deloitte-2022-genz-millennial-survey.pdf

3 https://www.mentalhealth.org.uk/sites/default/files/2022-06/MHF-Investing-in-Prevention-Report-Summary.pdf

4 https://www.mentalhealth.org.uk/explore-mental-health/a-z-topics/men-and-mental-health

5 https://www.ons.gov.uk/peoplepopulationandcommunity/wellbeing/articles/coronavirusanddepressioninadultsgreatbritain/julytoaugust2021

6 https://www.campaigntoendloneliness.org/the-facts-on-loneliness/

7 http://ccare.stanford.edu/uncategorized/connectedness-health-the-science-of-social-connection-infographic/

8 https://www.pulsetoday.co.uk/news/uncategorised/four-in-10-gps-regularly-see-lonely-patients-who-are-not-unwell/

9 https://thesleepmanifesto.com/downloads/the-sleep-manifesto-manifesto-january-2020_digital.pdf

10 https://www.ncbi.nlm.nih.gov/pmc/articles/PMC5175375/

11 https://jamanetwork.com/journals/jamapsychiatry/article-abstract/2780428

12 https://www.atlassian.com/blog/productivity/boredom-at-work-creativity-neuroscience?utm_source=newsletter-email&utm_medium=email&utm_campaign=work-life-blog-oct-13-2021_EML-10880&jobid=105217641&subid=1639856250

13 https://www.nvp.com/ceojourney-study/#tradeoffs-success

14 https://pubmed.ncbi.nlm.nih.gov/28126210/

15 https://www.sciencetheearth.com/uploads/2/4/6/5/24658156/2011_sakul-ku_the_impostor_phenomenon.pdf

16 https://journals.aom.org/doi/abs/10.5465/amj.2020.1627

17 https://www.pnas.org/content/early/2010/08/27/1011492107

18a https://greatergood.berkeley.edu/pdfs/GratitudePDFs/6Emmons-BlessingsBurdens.pdf

18b https://www.ncbi.nlm.nih.gov/pmc/articles/PMC1820947/

18c https://link.springer.com/article/10.1007/s10902-016-9735-z

18d https://www.sciencedirect.com/science/article/abs/pii/S0277953608000373 (page 131)

18e https://www.sciencedirect.com/science/article/abs/pii/S0191886910004769 (page 131)

18f https://journals.plos.org/plosone/article?id=10.1371/journal.pone.0160589

19 https://pubmed.ncbi.nlm.nih.gov/28527220/

20 https://www.medicalnewstoday.com/articles/what-percentage-of-the-human-body-is-water#avoiding-dehydration

21 https://alcoholchange.org.uk/alcohol-facts/fact-sheets/alcohol-statistics

22 https://pubmed.ncbi.nlm.nih.gov/30067939/

23 https://neuroimmunology.org.uk/

24 https://bmcmedicine.biomedcentral.com/articles/10.1186/s12916-017-0791-y

25 https://www.sciencedirect.com/science/article/abs/pii/S0169204619308163?via%3Dihub

26 https://pubs.acs.org/doi/10.1021/es305019p

27 https://www.projectxfactor.com/post/looking-at-fractals-reduce-stress-by-up-to-60

28 https://www.rcpsych.ac.uk/news-and-features/latest-news/detail/2021/05/05/rcpsych-declares-a-climate-and-ecological-emergency

29 https://www.nhs.uk/mental-health/self-help/guides-tools-and-activities/exercise-for-depression/

30 https://www.frontiersin.org/articles/10.3389/fpsyt.2013.00027/full

31 https://neurosciencenews.com/hippocampus-memory-anxiety-8784/

32 https://www.gov.uk/government/publications/prescribed-medicines-review-report/prescribed-medicines-review-summary

33 https://www.bmj.com/content/364/bmj.l1508

34 https://www.bbc.co.uk/news/health-47740396

35 https://evidence.nihr.ac.uk/alert/teenagers-use-of-antidepressants-is-rising-with-variations-across-regions-and-ethnic-groups/

36 https://www.theguardian.com/society/2021/jan/01/covid-antidepressant-use-at-all-time-high-as-access-to-counselling-in-england-plunges

37 https://www.ons.gov.uk/peoplepopulationandcommunity/wellbeing/articles/coronavirusanddepressioninadultsgreatbritain/june2020

RESOURCES

GENERAL

hubofhope.co.uk

nhs.uk

@dralexgeorge (Instagram)

youtube.com/DrAlexGeorge

George, Alex, *Live Well Every Day*, Aster, 2021

giveusashout.org

place2be.org.uk

nhs.uk/every-mind-matters

CONNECTION IS YOUR SUPERPOWER

ageuk.org.uk

doit.life/volunteer

campaigntoendloneliness.org

marmaladetrust.org

STRESS IS THE ENEMY

citizensadvice.org.uk

stepchange.org

themoneycharity.org.uk

MAKE FOOD YOUR FRIEND

bda.uk.com/resource/food-for-thought-the-role-of-nutrition-in-the-gut-brain-axis.html

nhs.uk/live-well/eat-well

bda.uk.com/food-health/food-facts.html

nutrition.org.uk

nhs.uk/better-health/drink-less

Bullmore, Edward, *The Inflamed Mind*, Picador, 2018

ALCOHOL SUPPORT

www.nhs.uk/better-health/drink-less

drinkaware.co.uk/tools

alcoholchange.org.uk

Drink Free Days app

NOMO app

Try Dry app

alcoholics-anonymous.org.uk

DON'T FORGET TO BREATHE

Headspace app

Insight Timer app

Calm app

nhs.uk/mental-health/self-help/tips-and-support/mindfulness

nhs.uk/mental-health/self-help/guides-tools-and-activities/breathing-exercises-for-stress

wimhofmethod.com

mrjamesnestor.com

IT'S GOOD TO TALK

nhs.uk/service-search/find-a-psychological-therapies-service

bacp.co.uk

psychotherapy.org.uk

bps.org.uk

bacp.co.uk/about-therapy/types-of-therapy

emdrassociation.org.uk

bsch.org.uk

nhs.uk/every-mind-matters

MENTAL-HEALTH CHARITIES

mind.org.uk

mentalhealth.org.uk

youngminds.org.uk

rethink.org

thecalmzone.net

HELPLINES

samaritans.org

supportline.org.uk

papyrus-uk.org

thecalmzone.net

switchboard.lgbt

giveusashout.org

spuk.org.uk

childline.org.uk

INDEX

AUTHOR'S ACKNOWLEDGEMENTS

I sit here writing this, reflecting over the last few years and everything that has happened, the highs and the lows. It's hard to get my head around the fact that *The Mind Manual* is my third book. I believe that no man is an island: I would not have been able to do any of the stuff that I've managed to do without the incredible people in both my personal and my professional life. What I am so grateful for is that my colleagues are also my friends, they are my second family. We stand shoulder to shoulder through the tough times as well as the good. To everyone at the Found Agency, thank you for everything, we do it together.

Stephanie Jackson needs a special mention – a true powerhouse and a person I really trust. I have enjoyed working with you and your team across these books. We have a lot to be proud of. Our shared drive and undeniable perfectionism have allowed us to create something that can and will make a difference. Thank you for making this all possible. We are helping people to live and thrive, not simply survive. What an incredible motivator that is. A huge thank you to everyone at Hachette who has given so much to make *The Mind Manual* the best it can possibly be. Your contributions will never be forgotten.

Over the last year, little Rolo Polo has joined the family, my beautiful furry friend. Although you will never be able to read this (that would be rather clever), I want to say thanks to you, my awesome pup. Since Rolo, we have also had a human addition to the family, my gorgeous goddaughter Cara Thomas. I am so excited to watch you grow and explore the world. Adam and Emma, you are wonderful and I'm so happy to be the third wheel in your marriage. Mam, Dad and Elliott, I love you and I continue to be so proud of you. We are closer than ever.

I want to close this by saying thank you to Abby Wagge, who has become my 'unflappable friend' (as Mam calls you). Although you work as my executive assistant, truly you are a little sister to me. I'm not going to say big sister, because your head will explode! Thank you to everyone who has worked with me over the last few years, to all of my friends and family. You are awesome and I love you all. Onwards we go.